Community-Based Participatory Research for Improved Mental Healthcare

Laura Weiss Roberts

Community-Based Participatory Research for Improved Mental Healthcare

A Manual for Clinicians and Researchers

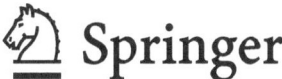 Springer

Laura Weiss Roberts
Department of Psychiatry & Behavioral Sciences
Stanford University School of Medicine
Palo Alto, CA, USA

ISBN 978-1-4614-5516-5   ISBN 978-1-4614-5517-2 (eBook)
DOI 10.1007/978-1-4614-5517-2
Springer New York Heidelberg Dordrecht London

Library of Congress Control Number: 2012951416

Printed on acid-free paper

Springer is part of Springer Science+Business Media (www.springer.com)

To Chris and Mark, outstanding
collaborators and loved friends
– Laura

To my parents, Rosemarie and
Bernhard, who personify
cooperation, mutuality, and respect
– Chris

To the memory of my good friend
and colleague, Lori Namyniuk,
who lived the spirit of CBPR
– Mark

To my husband, Jeff, and my
children, Adam, Kate, and Erin,
for their steadfast support and
love
– Jane

Foreword

Dharma Talks Under Three Moons

When I returned from Cambodia to my clinic in the San Francisco Bay area, I had many new ideas for clinical outcomes research for my Khmer mental health patients. In Siam Reap, I had seen the collaborations between mental health and Buddhist temples wherein the Khmer monks led mindfulness meditation groups for the reduction of anxiety symptoms in traumatized mental health patients with post-traumatic stress disorder. As the psychiatrist and clinical director of a Cambodian mental health program in San Jose, California, I wanted to implement a similar paradigm for the Khmer patients in my clinic and do community-based research on the outcomes. But to incorporate such a function, our clinic would need a Khmer Buddhist monk. This is a tall order in California. Through my culturally adept Cambodian clinician colleagues I was linked to the local Buddhist temple to pitch my idea of collaboration. The task would be to convince the abbot of the temple to lead mindfulness meditation groups for our clinic's patients.

We connected with people at the temple, and we gave an overview of the proposed clinical research project. The abbot invited me to join him for a "Dharma talk at the next new moon." I was eager to get started as soon as possible, but I waited.

On the next new moon, I went to the temple on that day and met the monks. The head monk sat with me on a mat before giant bodhisattva figures and burning incense and began a lecture on the Dharma. At the end of his lecture, he invited me to meditate with him. So I did. He taught some basic principles and we sat together in quiet meditation. When we finished he stood up and excused himself. I said, "Wait. Can we talk about the research project?" He replied, "Yes. We will talk when you come back at the quarter moon."

On the quarter moon, a week later, I came to the temple. Again, the head monk sat with me on a mat and began a lecture on the Dharma. Again, at the end of his lecture, he invited me to meditate with him. So I did. When we finished he stood up and excused himself. We had an exchange similar to the last visit regarding discussion of the research project. "We will talk when you come back at the full moon."

On the day of the full moon I returned. Rather than discuss research, I received a Dharma talk and a mindfulness meditation session with the head monk. This weekly pattern continued until the next new moon. At the end of that session, before he left I asked, "When can we talk about the research project?"

He smiled, gave a puzzled look, and responded, "We have been talking about the project for a full month now."

After another lunar cycle of weekly Dharma talks and mindfulness sessions, the monk's method had become clear to me. He had demanded my regular attendance to test my commitment to a partnership before he was willing to invest in the project. He had also used the regular meetings to establish a trust with me to satisfy his concern over whether I was dedicated to our mutual population. He was interested in working with me, but needed to make sure that my intention was true and that the work, in the end, would be for the benefit of the people in his community.

When the *third* new moon had come, we had our regular, weekly session. This time he did not get up to excuse himself. This time he said "Now we have completed a course in mindfulness meditation. How did you find it?"

"Quite enlightening," I replied truthfully.

"Good," he said smiling. "Now you understand. And now you understand what will be asked of all the people who take part in this project and you understand what they stand to gain through it. Now let us talk about your research."

Stanford, CA, USA   Daryn Reicherter

Preface

Ethical and Scientific Rationale
for Community-Based Participatory Research

Respect for Persons, Beneficence, and Justice are the principles that collectively form the ethical basis of human research (Department of Health, Education, and Welfare 1979). These three principles find expression in Community-Based Participatory Research, or CBPR — a systematic approach for engaging specially defined groups of people in a process of inquiry and social change. Central to CBPR is the demonstration of deep regard for the dignity and autonomy of individuals who constitute a "community" by virtue of residing in a certain geographic location; having a shared racial, ethnic, or cultural identity; or living with a particular illness. The intent of CBPR is to bring about good as defined by these communities in a manner that is characterized by emic understanding, mutuality, and fairness.

Fairness and mutualism have been elusive in the conduct of human studies, and together they represent perhaps the greatest ethical impetus for CBPR. Past exploitation of vulnerable populations — rather than fulfillment of the imperative for "equitable distribution of benefits and burdens in society" — is evidenced by, for example, the Tuskegee Syphilis Study, the Willowbrook Study, the Human Radiation Experiments, as well as hundreds if not thousands of other projects (Katz et al. 1972; Meslin 1996; Beecher 1966). In these studies, researchers were fundamentally dishonest in their dealings with participants. These exploitative projects "used" groups of people in society who were relatively disempowered for the principal benefit of more empowered groups of people, rather than for some other reason, such as the need to study vulnerable groups to address their own critical and neglected concerns. More recent research, though less obviously exploitative, has similarly damaged communities as significant or stigmatizing health issues have been discovered and the consequences of the findings not addressed (Foulks 1989). In these situations, characterized by asymmetry rather than mutualism, researchers attained their objectives of gaining new knowledge at the cost of groups of people without a voice who lacked the resources to repair the harm that was done by the research. By deliberately addressing fairness and mutualism CBPR endeavors to strengthen the justice commitment of human research.

The conduct of CBPR involves authentic participation of the community in identifying issues of scientific concerns that, in turn, derive from past empirical work or advances in theory or methods. Funding opportunities may also influence the questions undertaken for study, but only if in alignment with community and scientific considerations (Viswanathan et al. 2004; Minkler and Wallerstein 2008). CBPR is a process that involves co-learning. In CBPR, study design, recruitment and consent methods, measurements, interventions and/ or outcomes, data analysis, and interpretation are all shaped through an active and mutually respectful dialogue that unites community representatives and scientists. The findings of the study are shared quickly and directly with the community in many venues, and appropriate steps in the interests of the community are determined and enacted through coordinated CBPR research teams comprising community members and scientists in equal partnerships. New knowledge is shared with the scientific community and the public at large. Scientists and community representatives collaborate, with community members involved not only in the identification of the issues, but also the conceptualization, design, and conduct of the research. Community members have clear roles on the research team and are equal partners in the research endeavor. At each step of the way, methods support information-exchange, power-sharing, mutual decision-making, and accountability in the relationships among the members of the CBPR team, which always consists of scientists and community representatives.

Sound ethics leads to great science for society. By safeguarding the process of ethically sound research development, study implementation, and dissemination, science itself is rendered more rigorous, ecologically attuned, and accurate (Roberts 1999). As noted in a systematic review of the evidence for CBPR (Viswanathan et al. 2004), the Agency for Health Research and Quality argues that communities are more motivated to support the success of the research, more likely to accept the study approach and related resources, and more able to handle potentially sensitive issues in CBPR than in conventional research practice. The reviewers also point out that the measures used in CBPR tend to have greater reliability and validity, and the findings are more likely to be interpreted accurately by the research team. The true limitations to the generalizability of study findings are more likely to be clear. Moreover, results are culturally and socially "relevant" to the population and therefore more likely to serve as the basis for positive social change. The process of CBPR helps inspire trust in the scientific enterprise, which in turn allows for future collaborative, evidence-driven work, the progression of science, and the enhancement of community life. CBPR thus is ethically grounded, enriches science, and gives rise to positive societal impact as the new knowledge emerges from real-world settings.

CBPR is especially valuable in mental health research. Because people with neuropsychiatric diseases may become vulnerable to exploitation by virtue of the nature and the consequences of the illness process, additional safeguards—such as those found in CBPR—are essential to ensure their adequacy from an ethical perspective. Because neuropsychiatric diseases are poorly understood and have received relatively little study over the past 100 years, methods that allow these diseases to be researched and to have optimal impact are crucial. Because neuropsychiatric diseases are widespread and increasingly recognized for their global health impact, the imperative to use newly emerging techniques and methods to gain significant new knowledge is immense. Because of the sheer number and the vulnerability of stakeholders involved with the mental health community, a collaborative method is necessary and inexorable to ensure sound science. Finally, because neuropsychiatric diseases are often highly stigmatized, the greatest possible attention to the process of research is essential to minimize unintended harm to affected individuals and communities.

CBPR is effortful, but it builds capacity. This approach is defined by many conversations, many shared decisions, many compromises, many joys, and many consequences. The time arc for entering CBPR is different and slower than for other forms of research; yet, paradoxically, the translation to real-world benefit is accelerated and the sequence of science, once the collaborative community–researcher relationship is in place, progresses much more quickly. The effort inherent in CBPR is well rewarded in the capacity it creates for improving health outcomes and health research quality. CBPR generates capacity for public trust in science. As early career investigators become familiar with this mode of collaborative inquiry in the service of society, an exciting and entirely new capacity—for ethically sound and more rigorous and consequential science—is built. It is with these valuable capacities in mind that this handbook is offered.

Palo Alto, CA, USA   Laura Weiss Roberts

Authors

Laura Weiss Roberts, M.D., M.A.

Dr. Roberts serves as Chairman and the Katharine Dexter McCormick and Stanley McCormick Memorial Professor in the Department of Psychiatry and Behavioral Sciences at the Stanford University School of Medicine. She is an internationally recognized scholar in bioethics, psychiatry, medicine, and medical education. Dr. Roberts has received extensive scientific peer-reviewed funding from the National Institutes of Health, the Department of Energy, and private foundations to perform empirical studies of modern ethical issues in research, clinical care, and health policy, with a particular focus on vulnerable and special populations. Her work has led to advances in understanding of ethical aspects of physical and mental illness research, societal implications for genetic innovation, the role of stigma in health disparities, the impact of medical student and physician health issues, and optimal approaches to fostering professionalism in medicine. Dr. Roberts owns Terra Nova Learning Systems.

Christiane Brems, Ph.D., ABPP

At the time of this work, Dr. Brems served as Co-Director of the Center for Behavioral Health Research and Services at the University of Alaska Anchorage, Director of Clinical Training for the Joint Ph.D. Program in Clinical-Community Psychology at UAA, and Professor of Psychology at UAA. Dr. Brems has extensive research, teaching, clinical, and writing experience. Dr. Brems has authored books on a variety of clinical topics and published widely in professional journals. Her research and services grants have been funded by the National Institutes of Health and the Centers for Disorder Control and Prevention. Dr. Brems now is Dean for the School of Professional Psychology at Pacific University in Hillsboro, OR, and Professor Emerita at the University of Alaska Anchorage.

Mark E. Johnson, Ph.D.

At the time of this work, Dr. Johnson served as Co-Director of the Center for Behavioral Health Research and Services at the University of Alaska Anchorage and Professor of Psychology at UAA. His research has been funded through the National Institutes of Health and other federal and state agencies. Complementing his far-reaching research, teaching, and evaluation experience, Dr. Johnson is a licensed psychologist with extensive clinical experience with couples, adults, and supervision. He has published widely in professional journals and has presented at countless national and international conferences. Dr. Johnson now is a Research Professor in the College of Health Professions at Pacific University in Hillsboro, Oregon, and a Professor Emeritus at the University of Alaska Anchorage.

Jane Smikowski, M.A.

Ms. Smikowski earned a Master's Degree in Counseling at Marquette University in Milwaukee, Wisconsin, and is a member of Psi Chi Honors Society in Psychology. Ms. Smikowski has experience in counseling and advocating for families involved in the social welfare system, leading support and training for homeless women in positive parenting and personal empowerment, and providing college counseling services to young adults struggling with personal, mental health, academic, and career/vocational concerns. As Project Coordinator at Terra Nova Learning Systems, Ms. Smikowski has coordinated and contributed to the development of numerous National Institutes of Health-funded training and educational materials for a variety of audiences, including mental health providers, educators, and students.

Content Contributors

Catherine Bruss, B.A., and Renee Hesselbach, M.S., Terra Nova Learning Systems
Sarah Dewane, Ph.D., Providence Family Medicine Residency, Anchorage, Alaska

Video Reflection Contributors

Researchers

Gloria Eldridge, Ph.D., Associate Professor of Psychology, University of Alaska Anchorage
Carl M. Hild, Ph.D., M.S., Associate Professor, Alaska Pacific University, Anchorage, Alaska
Inna Rivkin, Ph.D., Assistant Professor of Psychology, University of Alaska Fairbanks
Tracy Speier, MPA, Public Health Researcher, Anchorage Alaska
Karen Ward, Ph.D., Professor and Director, Center for Human Development, University of Alaska Anchorage

Community Member

Cheryl Scott, Parent Navigator Training Coordinator, Anchorage, Alaska

About Terra Nova Learning Systems

This Community-Based Participatory Research resource was created by Terra Nova Learning Systems of Palo Alto, California, in conjunction with Drs. Brems and Johnson when they were directing the Center for Behavioral Health Research and Services (CBHRS) of the University of Alaska Anchorage. Terra Nova Learning Systems is dedicated to developing innovative educational materials that focus on scientific topics. Many of Terra Nova Learning System's projects relate to mental illness and substance abuse. Terra Nova endeavors to increase public awareness of the nature and importance of these disorders. The company's ultimate goal is to help lessen the burden and stigma experienced by persons living with mental disorders, increase awareness within the general public of important mental health concerns, and advance scientific capacities in society. Terra Nova Learning Systems has no relationship to the pharmaceutical industry.

This project has been funded in whole or in part with Federal funds from the National Institute of Mental Health, National Institutes of Health, Department of Health and Human Services, under Contract No. HHSN-271-2006-6-4092-C/ N44-MH-6-4092.

info@terranovalearning.com **I** 650-391-9565 **I** www.terranovalearning.com

Contents

Chapter 1
What Is Community-Based Participatory Research?

Welcome to *Community-Based Participatory Research for Improved Mental Healthcare: A Manual for Clinicians and Researchers*, a guide for medical, academic, and institutional professionals, as well as community leaders and advocates interested in pursuing a collaborative approach to research in which the daily realities of life that are unique to each community set the context for the study.

Over the last decade, the mental health profession has recognized the importance and value of local communities setting the context for research. Current advances in this field continue to support the premise that when the contextual realities of community life are a critically integral part of the research plan, process, and decision-making, the results of a study will *directly* address the needs of the target community (community needs influence all decision-making, producing study results that directly address the originally stated needs). As researchers conceptualize their community-based studies, community life on a personal level (i.e., the day-to-day realities of individual members) and a systemic level (i.e., social, political, economic, cultural, and environmental) must be considered. Only by developing a study from the community perspective will a researcher create a study that directly addresses the concerns of that community.

The *community-based participatory research* model, or CBPR, provides a framework for researchers and communities to partner in collaborative investigations of *community-identified* needs. Often, equality and respect within a CBPR partnership begin when community

L.W. Roberts, *Community-Based Participatory Research for Improved Mental Healthcare*, DOI 10.1007/978-1-4614-5517-2_1,
© Springer Science+Business Media New York 2013

representatives contribute to naming the research question. Community input and perspective are held in highest regard by the research team throughout the life of the study. CBPR centers on an ongoing, respectful, and equitable partnership between researchers and the community with a shared vision of co-creating positive change within the community studied.

The CBPR Process

The CBPR process begins with the identification of a specific concern within a community. This concern can be named by the community itself or determined in collaboration with the research team. Often, communities will seek out a research team to investigate a self-identified problem. Alternatively, a research team may become aware of a local issue, and approach a neighboring community to offer their assistance. No matter what unique circumstances bring the partners together, the following general principles guide both the project work and the partnership.

Researchers must be respectful of the culture, hierarchy of power, gatekeepers, and other factors when entering a community. They must find ways to engage with its members, develop mutual trust, and work as partners in all phases of the study—formulating the research question, developing the methodology, addressing day-to-day problems that arise, guiding outcomes, disseminating findings, and developing appropriate interventions.

At every step along the way, community partners are highly valued and respected for the unique perspectives they bring to the project. Community partners are experts in community life, and as experts they bring invaluable information to the project. Viewing each step of the study through the community lens is critical for its success. Researchers must consistently strive to maintain an appropriate balance of influence and responsibility among researchers and community partners to ensure that the study is conducted *with* a community rather than *on* a community.

Throughout the life of a study, the CBPR process is cyclical, iterative, and dynamic. It is continually and collaboratively adjusted and refocused in response to new knowledge that is discovered during the process.

The Research Partnership

A CBPR research team can include professionals from within or outside the community, such as physicians, psychologists, educators, social workers, mental health and substance abuse counselors, nurses, and other behavioral healthcare specialists. Community partners might also include individuals living with mental illness, their family members and caregivers, and other community leaders and advocates. The most important goal when gathering a group of community partners is to be sure that all voices are heard—even those that have been silent or marginalized in the past.

The voice of the community must come first in determining both the questions to address and ultimately the solutions to those questions.

Steven Adelsheim, M.D.
Professor of Psychiatry, Pediatrics, & Family/Community Medicine, University of New Mexico School of Medicine

Determining When CBPR Is the Right Approach

A crucial question for any researcher is: When is CBPR is the best approach to take? Due to its flexible nature, community-based participatory research can be easily adapted to a wide variety of situations. However, despite its many advantages it is not always the best approach for a given research project. Important variables should be considered before engaging in a CBPR study. These variables are discussed in detail throughout this book. Because no two research projects are alike, this book is not designed to be a "how to" manual for CBPR, but rather it is intended to provide researchers with a guide in thinking through many of the elements that are critical to a successful CBPR study.

After completing this book, research professionals should be well equipped to determine the appropriateness and value of conducting a CBPR study with a community. This book is designed to provide researchers with the information they need to answer the following basic questions:

- Will the community as well as the research team benefit from a CBPR approach?
- Can the community and research team find unity in purpose and process?
- Is the community prepared to take on the responsibilities of a research partnership?
- Does the research team have the time and dedication required for a CBPR study, including time spent before, during, and after the study?
- Does the research team possess the skills required to conduct a CBPR study?

After reading this book, the researcher will be better able to determine answers to these questions, and to determine whether CBPR is the best approach. Over the course of any CBPR project, it is crucial that researchers keep their work focused primarily on benefit to the community. That is, the ultimate goals of CBPR should always be to generate information that will ultimately benefit the community, and support capacity-building of community partners.

The goal of *Community-Based Participatory Research for Improved Mental Healthcare* is to educate mental health researchers on the principles and processes of this often-complex research approach, and to provide access to tools needed to conduct successful CBPR studies.

Researcher Reflection

What research characteristics are a good fit for CBPR?

In community-based research, or participatory research, you're looking at turning over a lot of control to other people. It's not like doing lab research where you have this notion that "I'm

(continued)

going to control all the sources of variability and I'm going to design how the study is going to occur." With community research you're working with other people who come from a much different perspective, so you need to be flexible, you need to have a respect for other ways of knowing, and you need to have a respect for the people that you're working with. Rather than looking at people as subjects, you have to look at them as collaborators. And you have to do more than look at them, you have to actually feel that they are collaborators and know that they are collaborators. I think it takes a particular kind of scientist to be able to do this kind of work well.

Excerpted from an interview with Gloria Eldridge, Ph.D., Associate Professor of Psychology, University of Alaska Anchorage

Book Outline

In the five chapters that follow, discussion of the CBPR process will be framed by these questions:

Chapter 2: Background Preparation for the CBPR Process

- What is important about community participation?
- What are the goals of the research relationship with the community?
- How are communities chosen—scientifically, ethically, and collaboratively—when the research originates outside of the community?
- What is the relevant history, and where are the potential sources of trust and mistrust?
- How does the research staff prepare for the relationships and responsibilities of community participatory research?
- What are the practical resource issues?

Chapter 3: Beginning Partnerships with Communities

- Who are the key leaders and natural wise persons with whom trustworthiness and integrity must be demonstrated?
- When and how do researchers approach a community?

- What information is appropriate to share about the scientific questions, the methodology, and the anticipated *risks* and *benefits* to the community and to individual participants?
- How do researchers figure out ways to minimize risk to the community?
- How are community advisory boards developed, and how will healthy, effective functioning be facilitated?
- How should values conflicts and disagreements be addressed?

Chapter 4: Finding Common Ground Within the Partnership

- How do researchers determine the values and needs of the community?
- How are implicit concerns expressed?
- How do partners find common ground on differing goals and preferences?
- What are the processes for dealing with conflicts and disagreements on an ongoing basis?
- What if the partnership fails?
- What ethical safeguards does the community need or want?
- What are the jurisdiction issues?

Chapter 5: Sustaining the Partnership

- How are day-to-day issues addressed?
- How is the equality of all partners maintained throughout the process?
- How are all partners kept informed of process and progress?
- How are community advisory boards maintained?
- How are major changes in the "ground rules" addressed and communicated?

Chapter 6: Evaluating the Partnership and Enhancing Future Successes

- How are study results used in ways that are acceptable to all?
- How is the relationship sustained when the work of the research study is finished?
- How and why have reflection and debriefing become essential activities?
- How is the success of the process involved in project implementation evaluated from the perspectives of all stakeholders?

Community Materials

The content in this book is enhanced by the following materials:

Researcher reflections*. We have provided quotes gleaned from real-world researchers as they reflect on their experiences with *community-based participatory research*. Presented in callout boxes and with some reflections available in online video interview clips, these statements provide key insights into changes in thinking, adjustments to prior assumptions about self or others, and ways in which researchers must rethink their typical processes to respectfully join with community partners. These quotes are meant to remind readers that ongoing self-reflection is critical to achieving successful CBPR.

Community member reflections*. We have provided reflections from community members sharing comments and opinions about CBPR. Placed in callout boxes within topic pages, with some reflections available in online video interview clips, these statements present important perspectives on the research process and remind researchers to gather community perspectives and insights at each stage of the process.

Case studies. A variety of real-world CBPR case examples can be found at the end of each chapter. Each case study underscores important topics and concepts discussed in the chapter content. Some of the case studies relate to noteworthy CBPR projects that have been conducted (references provided).

Glossary. A full listing with definitions of important CBPR terms can be found at the back of the book.

*For video versions of these features, go to http://www.terra-novalearning.com and enter the following:
username: community
password: outreach

*Community Outreach Kit**

With the purchase of this book, research professionals can access online outreach materials for use when establishing a CBPR study within a community. Materials can be downloaded and printed "as is" from the website listed at the end of this section. Or a researcher may opt to re-create these layouts in any fashion—adding local artwork, terminology, and information unique to a particular research community. Color copies of all print materials can be ordered from the Terra Nova Learning website for an additional fee. Materials listed below that are followed by (S) are also available in Spanish.

The Community Outreach Kit includes:

Researcher guide. A handy, concise checklist containing salient information to guide research work with communities. Relationship-building, conflict resolution, and self-reflection strategies are among the areas of focus. A copy of the Research Guide can be found in Appendix A.

*Community Brochure**.* An easy-to-understand booklet designed to provide community members with basic information about CBPR (e.g., can be used at the first community meeting, during discussions with community leaders, as a guide for local research partners who will assist in a project). Layout is set up to be printed two-sided, and then folded in half and stapled down the middle, but can also be printed as a single-sided piece. Printing instructions appear in the Facilitator Guide. Sample pages of the Community Brochure can be found in Appendix B. (S)

CBPR slide presentation. A slide show that corresponds to the Community Brochure, for researcher use during small and large group meetings, or for one-on-one discussions. Available in PowerPoint and PDF formats. (S)

Facilitator guide. A guide to assist researchers in conducting initial community meetings. Contains general group facilitation tips and background information on basic CBPR concepts. The Table of Contents and sample pages from the Facilitator Guide can be found in Appendix C.

*Posters**.* Engaging, customizable posters for a variety of purposes (e.g., for meeting announcements, use as a community handout, display in meeting rooms). A sample poster can be found in Appendix D. (S)

Newspaper ad**. A customizable newspaper ad template for study recruitment or announcement purposes. A sample newspaper ad can be found in Appendix E. (S)

Stationery. Blank letterhead for multiple uses (e.g., letters, press releases, additional handouts).

> *To access these materials online, go to http://www.terra-novalearning.com and enter the following:
> **username: community**
> **password: outreach**

**These PDF documents contain editable fields for electronic entry of research-related information (name of study, contact name, and phone number, etc.). If your version of Adobe Acrobat does not allow entry of text into PDFs, information may be added in pen, using a preprinted label, or in any other fashion.

Chapter 2
Background Preparation for the CBPR Process

Upon completion of **Chapter 2: Background Preparation for the CBPR Process**, the reader will be able to:

- Describe how CBPR differs from traditional research.
- Summarize the primary issues associated with defining and identifying a community.
- Explain the importance of joining a community in advance of conducting the work of a CBPR project.

Introduction

Community-based participatory research centers on a highly respectful collaboration between a professional research team and the members of a study community. It is a process that relies heavily on researchers effectively engaging with local people and employing local knowledge and experience to help create meaningful research that *directly* benefits the study community. By viewing an issue through the community's lens, researchers gain a deeper understanding of local mental health concerns as defined by the community and are better able to conduct research that may lead to appropriate and relevant interventions.

The participatory research process uses an ecological approach, which recognizes that many individual, social, political, economic, cultural, and environmental systems that are in place within a community can influence the availability and access of its members to

L.W. Roberts, *Community-Based Participatory Research for Improved Mental Healthcare*, DOI 10.1007/978-1-4614-5517-2_2,
© Springer Science+Business Media New York 2013

mental health resources. The CBPR process considers how the inter-actions of these systems can contribute to a community's mental health concerns and recognizes the value of looking at this "bigger picture" when considering any community interventions.

Chapter 2 of *Community-Based Participatory Research for Improved Mental Healthcare* focuses on the preparatory groundwork that is critical to a successful CBPR project. This chapter underscores some of the work that must be conducted in advance of beginning a CBPR project including important relationship-building steps that are critical in the early stages of a study.

Researcher Reflection

What is the recipe for successful CBPR?

Community research is, and I probably won't get the propor-tions quite right, one part science, two parts relationship, three parts trust, and probably two and a half parts long-term com-mitment. So you have to bring all of those things in and rela-tionship and trust are certainly critical aspects because without those, any amount of science that you know and any amount of wonderful ideas that you may have are just not going to get done. It's all about relationships and trustworthiness.

Excerpted from a video interview with Gloria Eldridge, Ph.D., Associate Professor of Psychology, University of Alaska Anchorage

What Is Important About Community Participation?

When community partners "weigh-in" early in project planning, researchers are certain to "start where the people are." By continuing to reach out to community partners throughout the process, research-ers will stay focused on benefit to the community and not risk turning the study toward their professional interests. The researcher–commu-nity partnership sets the stage for valuable co-learning to occur. Just as the community learns from the scientific knowledge and expertise of the research team, so too do the researchers gain valuable knowledge from their community partners, who are *resident experts* on local community life. Since participatory research is conducted in the community, with community members, results from the study will specifically address locally relevant issues and will provide benefits uniquely tailored to a particular community.

Defining Community

Community-based research recognizes "community" as an identity. Members have both individual and collective identification (such as membership in a family, position in a social network, or identity linked to a geographic location). Many of these identities are socially constructed, and are created, changed, and strengthened through various levels of social interaction within communities. Community identity can be defined by established norms and values, existing systems and levels of influence and power, and common interests and needs. A community is often defined as a specific geographic neighborhood, or it may be a subgroup within that location. Community might also be defined by an ethnic, faith-based, or age-related group with a strong sense of common identity and situation. An urban neighborhood may contain several overlapping communities within its aggregate population.

Example:
John, employed by the local municipality, said that his current communities include his family, the city in which he lives and works, the elementary school community where his children go to school and where he is an active PTA member, a local athletic club in which he has been a long-time member, the long-time friends with whom John likes to socialize, the neighborhood in which he lives, the political party in which he is active, his church community, the country in which he pays taxes, and the state in which he lives. John is also a member of a support group for parents of children with developmental disabilities and a local community service group.

Researchers often face challenges in defining and identifying "community," but it is an essential first step upon which others in the study will be built. Identifying the study community enables researchers to begin to understand the social structure, including power hierarchies that are in place, such as who are the influential community leaders, spokespeople, or gatekeepers; who will likely provide reliable/less reliable information; is there a history of research wrongdoing and resulting mistrust; who may choose to actively limit/promote certain community voices or perspectives; and how might one reach the community's most hidden members?

Benefits of Community Participation

Recent developments in research methodology and ethics, supported by a more broad belief of what constitutes "expert knowledge," confirm the value of community perspectives and opinions as crucial elements of the research process. Including community input into each step of the process significantly increases levels of research validity and generalizability in the study, when that input comes from a group of partners who bring new perspectives and diverse skills, backgrounds, and experiences to the table. Collaboration between CBPR partners blends a broad scope of "ways of knowing" to inform ethical, scientifically rigorous research that is designed specifically to benefit the community under study.

Example:
A graduate-level student researcher attending a local university reflected on the process after working with a nearby community. "Our first task was really not to do anything at all. We spent the first few months listening… just listening to what the people of the community had to say. We listened as they told us what was really important to them, and we heard the things that they believed were possible. That was so helpful in shaping our project." While conducting the study, the team began to understand that when a group of people (researchers and community members) bring commitment and unique experience to the table, and take time to develop trust, then the ownership among the group is increased, power is shared and everyone feels important and respected.

In addition to contributing to the richness and meaning of the research study, community participation contributes a necessary element to the co-learning process. Many marginalized populations have not previously held enough power to either name or address their own mental health issues. But as knowledge is gained and transferred between partners in a community-based study, so too are skills, capacity, and feelings of empowerment. The participatory research process may address some of the power hierarchies that have occurred in the past between the researcher and participants by creating a

> *Involvement of community partners should begin when an idea is first being developed. Involvement at every stage decreases misunderstandings, builds trust, and results in unique outcomes that are culturally appropriate to the communities they represent.*
>
> Cheryl Gore-Felton, Ph.D.,
> Professor and Associate Chair, Department of Psychiatry and Behavioral Sciences, Stanford University

process of shared power. When conducting a CBPR study, critical importance is placed on respectful information-sharing, mutual decision-making, sharing of resources, and ongoing support among all members of the partnership. As team members (researchers and community members) become more invested in the study, feelings of ownership, commitment, and capacity for real and lasting community change are shared by all partners.

Researcher Reflection

What is community?

I would define community as the people who are impacted by your study. So if you're devising a program on intervention for people affected by HIV, you want to reach out to people affected by HIV. If you're trying to develop a program that might be a later implemented into an AIDS service organization, it's important to include people who are at those AIDS service organizations. Also bring in other people who understand the issues and who might provide services, for example, for people living with AIDS: health services, churches and other faith-based organizations. It's important to include a wide variety of people from the community so you're not getting just one viewpoint. It's hard to define community because there are so many people who could be impacted by a program and not everyone will have the same kinds of reactions to it.

Excerpted from a video interview with Inna Rivkin, Ph.D., Assistant Professor of Psychology, University of Alaska Fairbanks

What Are the Goals of the Research Relationship with the Community?

As the study progresses, a dynamic interplay of participation, cooperation, influence, self-reflection, and learning occurs among the research partners. In order to maintain an equitable balance of power, trust, and respect among all team members, professional researchers may have to adjust their long-held views of research in which, traditionally, they maintained complete control of the study. In CBPR, the traditional research approach must be modified to include community members as respected research partners with meaningful input and important decision-making power.

Example:
Members of a local community were willing to make a strong commitment to a research partnership with a local university only if the academic researchers demonstrated a sincere appreciation and respect for community partners' knowledge and experience. The community had past experience with university researchers who saw themselves as "experts" and who undervalued and even discounted the community members' input about issues and needs. The potential community partners were also concerned about university researchers' tendencies to present their points from a theoretical perspective, making it difficult to relate to real issues and daily community life.

The relationship between the community and the scientific research team extends beyond the traditional parameters of research work and should include the following.

University researchers must approach community partnerships with respect, humility, and recognition of the value of each community voice.

Steven Adelsheim, M.D.,
Professor of Psychiatry, Pediatrics, & Family/Community Medicine, University of New Mexico School of Medicine

---

Research Relationship Goals

- *Maintaining a truly participatory process*—All partners in the process should be mindful of the difference between involvement and participation. Community <u>involvement</u> suggests merely *inclusion* at some level in the process, while, in the case of CBPR, <u>participation</u> implies a somewhat *equal level of effort and influence* between researchers and community partners. Equity within the partnership often includes mutual collaboration or agreement on strategies for identifying needs, developing the study methodology, implementing strategies, gathering and recording data, disseminating results, and implementing change within the community.

- *Upholding equity of power, cooperation, engagement, and respect for all partners*—Traditional research has long held the view that participants are passive subjects. Community-based research challenges this viewpoint by redefining "expert knowledge" and by committing to a dynamic process of information-sharing which helps build capacity among all partners. By assigning great value to many diverse perspectives, this process takes advantage of the synergistic relationship that occurs between the scientific knowledge of researchers and the experiential, practical knowledge of community members. New knowledge created by the partners within the process of the study is consistently integrated back into the ongoing work of the study to inform action in a continuous feedback loop that lasts throughout the life of the project.
- *Building on strengths and resources within the community*—CBPR seeks out and builds upon strengths and resources that are in place within a community. The process dictates the incorporation of individual strengths, networks of relationships, organizational resources, and systems of power and respect into the conduct of mental health research. Although it is important to understand the community's needs and strengths early on, these topics are likely dynamic and will require ongoing attention and monitoring.
- *Recognizing that the research partnership is an ongoing co-learning experience*—Both researchers and community partners recognize that they learn from each other and that this learning process will continue throughout the life of the project. Because of the collaborative nature of the CBPR process, historically marginalized groups that have not been previously involved in identifying or addressing their own mental health needs are heard and the value of their contributions is recognized. Researchers understand the importance of community input, the value of community capacity-building, and that they have a great deal to learn from their partners.

- *Appreciating the cyclic nature of participatory research*—All research goals are not necessarily defined at the beginning of work with a community. As diverse perspectives are heard and new insights are gained, experimental methods and processes are likely to need adjustment and refinement to reflect this new knowledge. As partners share their views and opinions, critical self-reflection and meaningful dialogue among the partners create emerging knowledge that can be used to effectively inform project work and facilitate additional insights. As the work of the study progresses, researchers may need to develop support mechanisms to keep community partners engaged in the process, help them debrief new knowledge and experiences, and help them integrate what has been learned into their work.
- *Building bridges from what is to what is possible*—When individuals with diverse perspectives work together equitably, new light may be shed on community issues. When insights from a diverse group of people are shared, all members of the group begin to conceptualize new ways of thinking and of creating bridges from what is to what is possible. CBPR supports shifting emphasis from highly structured, clinical research to collaborative, dynamic research—building on real life experiences. When issues are defined by the community, and when community partners help guide the study, authentic, useful, targeted interventions and treatment options that truly "fit" the community are an attainable goal.

These goals take into consideration that a relationship between the researchers and the community exists in *advance* of the work of the project. When researchers begin a project in response to a funding solicitation, there may not be adequate time to develop the feelings of trust and cooperation within the community. Beginning a new relationship is not something that can be successfully accomplished during the typical 6-week grant-writing period. CBPR researchers need to work with communities in which they have an existing relationship already in place prior to starting a project. Perhaps it may be necessary to develop and sustain relationships months or years in advance of applying for grant money. Also, an established relationship with a community will help researchers more fully understand the community's needs within the context of its culture and values. This relationship-building groundwork may involve many hours of unpaid service and community involvement, and its importance to successful CBPR cannot be overlooked or overemphasized.

How Are Communities Chosen—Scientifically, Ethically, and Collaboratively—When the Research Originates Outside of the Community?

Researchers face significant challenges in their efforts to identify and define a study community. As stated in the previous section, if researchers have a strong relationship with a larger, local community, they will be better attuned to subgroups within the community and to specific mental health needs within those subgroups. Potential community partners may also be categorized into broad groups, such as those defined by geographic area, cultural heritage, religious affiliation, age, language, gender, race, ethnicity, or mental health concern. In other cases, the social contexts of members' lives may define more subtle communities.

It is crucial to solicit input from community members regarding "who" constitutes a community and what its main characteristics are. Researchers may define a community one way, whereas local members may disagree and define it in other ways. Defining a community without gathering input from respected community members may lead to misidentification of some of the most important or most marginal stakeholders. Some definitions of community may take into consideration only stakeholders with power and influence and may overlook marginalized members. It is the responsibility of the research team to have a relationship in which they can be certain that a broad scope of community perspectives and influence is represented.

Example:
Local university researchers studying homeless youth understood, early on, the diversity of this population. Their initial contact with the community occurred in areas where street youth were known to congregate. The team later moved out to other areas as they learned more about the homeless youth culture. They learned that most of the homeless youth congregating in the bus station were relatively new to street life, and behaviorally were more likely to engage in prostitution, contrasted by those more experienced in street life, who generally resided in downtown locations and were reportedly more heavily involved in drug dealing. Had the researchers assumed that the group of homeless youth found at

the bus station was representative of all street youth, they would have failed to gain an adequate understanding of the community and they might have recruited partners and volunteers from a very limited, unrepresentative group.

Methods of choosing a research community will vary in any given partnership, depending on current relationships, who is naming the research topic, how the community is defined, who defines it, and who joins the team as representatives of the community. Recognizing that no simple answer or strategy exists, researchers need to consider several questions.

Partnership in community-based participatory research presumes that the researcher and the community partner each has something to offer. If that presumption is correct, the expectations should be clarified. If that presumption is incorrect, the 'partnership' should be reconsidered altogether.

Daryn Reicherter, M.D.,
Clinical Associate Professor, Department of Psychiatry and Behavioral Sciences, Stanford University

---

Considerations When Selecting a Community for a Research Study

- What are the criteria that describe the community?
- Who defined the community?
- Who represents this community?
- How are boundaries of the community decided?
- What is the history of the community?
- Are partners involved as individuals, groups, or representatives of community-based organizations (CBOs)?
- Do the community representatives adequately represent the overall community in terms of class, income, gender, race, age, ethnicity, influence, etc.?
- Do individuals or representatives have the time and resources to serve on committees, attend meetings, and review information as needed for the duration of the study?
- Has the community initiated the research process?
- Is the community open to the research process?

- What are some barriers that might complicate development or completion of a community-based research project?
- Is the issue one that divides the community?
- Are there community members who may obstruct research efforts?

Community research is far more demanding on researchers than traditional research. It requires a certain type of person with professional training, and also a mindset and personality that values, and is inspired by, human relationships, motivation, and purpose.

What Is the Relevant History, and Where Are the Potential Sources of Trust and Mistrust?

Researchers need to take the time to develop a complete and thorough understanding of the local community members with regard to past history, current circumstances, and future visions. Engaging with and listening to a variety of community voices will help create knowledge and appreciation that together help form the basis for successful CBPR.

In traditional research, the community typically is not involved in designing the research project. Also, if the project runs into problems (for example, when a study takes a long time or costs too much money), community members, who have invested their time and energy, may find that they are left without a resolution to the issue that was studied or challenges that were identified. Further, traditional studies have occurred within communities without the participation, input, or knowledge of community leaders. Not surprisingly, such approaches have led to numerous cases of researchers collecting data and then sharing the data with the scientific community or public at large without first discussing and interpreting the findings with the community itself. Even worse, findings may not be disseminated in a manner that affects meaningful change or improvements to the community studied, or may cast a negative light on the community when shared with a broad audience.

Over time, as problems such as these have occurred, communities have rightfully become suspicious of researchers and have become unwilling to cooperate with them. CBPR responds to these issues by requiring that researchers engage community members and develop a relationship in advance of starting a project. This is the first, critical step in building a foundation of trust from which to establish a mutually beneficial, equitable research partnership. During the process of creating this foundation, the researchers must have a clear understanding of the community's values, needs, and expectations. They must *not* make assumptions based on their own knowledge or expertise, even if such knowledge is grounded in community-based work elsewhere.

By taking an open-minded approach, an atmosphere of collaboration, empowerment, and respect becomes possible. As trusting partnerships are formed, community members may decide that it is beneficial for them to invest the effort and resources needed for a given project. However, researchers must recognize that reaching this level of trust takes time. It is not uncommon for researchers to take up to a year to establish an environment in which community members feel safe and are trusting. Rushing this part of the process could result in the community's disinterest in beginning a study or pulling out from a study that has been started, particularly if it has experienced prior research wrongdoing. The following are some common potential sources of community mistrust of which researchers should be aware:

- Small, close-knit communities often have a basic mistrust of outsiders in general. Close-knit communities often display characteristics that include independence and self-sufficiency. They commonly access help through an informal system of neighbors and friends, and may not be interested in or trustful of the benefits of scientific studies or outside health experts.
- Data from traditional research may have, in the past, been used inappropriately, out of context, or for financial or professional gain for the researchers with no obvious or tangible benefit to the community.
- Research findings may not have always been interpreted and used or shared in a manner acceptable to the community.
- Previous inappropriate or disrespectful public reporting of research results may have led to destructive notoriety or stigmatization of communities or populations.
- Conflict with past research partners may have arisen as a result of dual agendas and goals (e.g., furthering the researcher's career versus identified community needs).

- Researchers may have "used" communities in traditional studies without providing adequate information about the purpose of the study or how the results would be used.
- Communities may have felt victimized by being "over-researched" in regard to specific mental health issues.
- Researchers may have promised in good faith that they would remain a visible presence in the community after a study was finished, but later pulled back from this commitment.

For many of us, we are not the first 'outsiders' to go into a community... it is important to understand the history and experiences of a particular community with regard to working with researchers because time may have to be dedicated to 'undoing deeds of the past' to build collaborative and trusting relationships. Taking a stance of compassion and understanding is essential in helping communities heal.

Cheryl Gore-Felton, Ph.D.,
Professor and Associate Chair, Department of Psychiatry and Behavioral Sciences, Stanford University

Researcher Reflection

What advice would you offer a researcher entering a community that's been harmed in the past?

When there's harm that has been done by studies that violated the trust of the community, I think it's really critical to first rebuild that trust, and to acknowledge that it will take time to rebuild the trust. Also, you need to spend facetime in the community so that people can see past your behavior and know that you're somebody who can be trusted. You must also show openness and show how your research is different than the research that might have preceded yours that didn't have that openness and integration of community perspectives.

Excerpted from a video interview with Inna Rivkin, Ph.D., Assistant Professor of Psychology, University of Alaska Fairbanks

You have to let people decide for themselves what they need. A well-respected doctor came to a community thinking he had already figured out what they needed to do. He meant well, but what he had planned would never work *and* it wasn't what the community needed *or* wanted.

How Does the Research Staff Prepare for the Relationships and Responsibilities of Community Participatory Research?

When conducting participatory research with communities, researchers may need to alter their concepts of what constitutes scientific research. Whereas traditional research is a highly structured, linear process, CBPR is a cyclical, dynamic, and iterative process where new knowledge created during the process informs ongoing project work. In traditional research, a study is conducted *on* participants, but in participatory research, participants are partners, and project work is conducted *with* them. The fact that community-based research goals are not always completely defined at the beginning of the work often challenges conventionally trained researchers. Individuals trained in traditional research methodologies *must* invest time to understand the participatory process before beginning a CBPR study, and must be committed to accepting and employing the principles and practices of participatory research.

In the CBPR process, the personal characteristics, behaviors, and activities of the research staff as scientists *and* human beings become more salient than in traditional research (in which investigators maintain distance from the people and phenomena under study). The following are suggestions to assist research team members as they begin to align themselves with a community.

Guidelines for Entering Communities

- *Become involved*—Prior to beginning the actual work of the project, the research staff should establish roots in the community. Research staff members can become visible, for example, by participating in community-sponsored events or volunteering their time to local organizations. By actively joining the community, the research staff has the opportunity to identify and evaluate any preconceived ideas or impressions they have about the community. In fact, each community has its own personality and set of circumstances; there is no such thing as a *typical* community.

- *Study social settings including levels of power and influence*—Researchers must gain experiential knowledge of the social structures that exist, and refrain from making uninformed predictions about those settings. For example, community gatekeepers can add credibility and support to a project, and they can also erect barriers to the community and its members. In one community a gatekeeper refused access to her friends claiming that they "aren't interested in that sort of thing." However, when these individuals were contacted through different routes, they were very interested in becoming involved. If the researchers had not pursued various means of recruitment, they would have missed out on a set of rich and unique perspectives and narratives. By becoming familiar with the community's systems and structure of social hierarchy and power, researchers will recognize when they must respect those systems, such as in certain ethnic families. For example, elders in Latino families are central members of the community. Family members are very protective of their patriarchs, and researchers must respect the family hierarchy.

- *Remain open to differences*—Throughout all interactions, researchers must continually remain open to the realities of community life, without judging those realities, and resist the impulse to change them. It is critically important for researchers to learn the community's ideas about boundaries of acceptable values, behavior, and lifestyle. As the partnership is forming, differences such as speech, dress, beliefs, and values must be accepted and respected by both the community partners and the research team.

CBPR researchers often struggle to maintain a balance between retaining their identity and role in the partnership and consistently respecting without judgment the unique contributions and situation of community partners. Collaborative partnering with communities means that researchers have been invited into the personal views, circumstances, and lives of community members. Strict adherence to ethical principles and unwavering respect of the community as individual members and as a whole are essential. Protection of the community must consistently remain a top priority for the research team.

Given the dynamic and cyclic nature of CBPR, research teams should remain in close contact with their Institutional Review Boards (IRBs). As a study progresses, and new information is evaluated by the team of study partners, research plans are often adjusted many times. Research teams must be vigilant about communicating protocol changes to their IRB.

Researcher Attributes That Help Ensure CBPR Success

- Flexible, respectful, and nonjudgmental attitude
- Recognition of one's own perspectives and of personal limitations, assumptions, and biases
- Emotional stability to undertake the complexity, unpredictability, diversity, and conflict inherent in CBPR work
- Commitment to equity with research partners
- Excellent group process skills
- Training in cultural sensitivity
- A high degree of political awareness
- Versatility and openness to new ways of knowing

Researcher Reflection

What is the difference between traditional and participatory research?

The difference is the notion of collaboration, relationships, trust, flexibility, and the idea that as a scientist you are bringing a somewhat limited set of tools into an environment where other people have a good sense of what the problem is and have a sense of what the solution is. You're bringing some tools to bear on that problem but you are not, by any means, the main event. And it's easy when you are a researcher to think that, "I've got this wonderful idea...I've got this methodology...I've got this way of approaching it, and if I can just get subjects or participants in my study then everything will be wonderful. But with community-based research the relationship is very different and you kind of need to bury your initial notion.

Excerpted from a video interview with Gloria Eldridge, Ph.D., Associate Professor of Psychology, University of Alaska Anchorage

What Are the Practical Resource Issues?

A number of practical resource issues must be taken into account in order to support a successful CBPR study. The research team must consider intangible resources such as time, energy, and commitment throughout the life of the project, as well as tangible resources such as physical barriers to participation and staff resources to conduct the study.

The complexities of establishing a CBPR study may exceed those of traditional research, due in large part to participation barriers that exist in many communities. In addition to the difficulties of gaining entry and acceptance in the community, other issues may arise that require ongoing and careful attention.

Potential Barriers to Participation

- Transportation difficulties, often due to geographically remote locations, that may interfere with representative community sampling
- Language and educational barriers that make scientific or technical information difficult to understand
- Close-knit communities with members who possess an inherent mistrust of outsiders
- Mental health-related issues that prevent involvement in social and other activities and leading to social isolation, rendering already marginalized community members inaccessible to researchers
- Communities that are disproportionately composed of individuals who belong to marginalized age groups (e.g., elders, children), ethnic minorities, or other historically marginalized groups
- Community members who do not have access to adequate health care, particularly those in remote areas
- Lack of anonymity in some communities, along with the stigma associated with mental illness, preventing treatment-seeking or study-related involvement
- Shortages of community mental health professionals, causing lack of diagnosis of mental health issues
- Poverty leading to difficulties in affording adequate health care

In addition, the amount of time community members are able to commit to a research study can often be a significant obstacle. Although research staff may be able to dedicate numerous hours to a study, community partners may be more limited as they are also involved with activities and commitments of their daily lives. Community agencies involved in the study that plan to rely on staff involvement must consider the amount of time staff members will be expected to contribute to the work of the study in addition to their daily responsibilities. The research team must be realistic about the time commitment they expect from community partners. It is important to remember that most, if not all, decisions regarding a study are made in consultation with all partners. Researchers must not underestimate the importance of having detailed discussions with partners about all levels of expectations in regard to the work of the study. This is fundamental to the collaborative process. Changes, adjustments, and evaluation of progress all require group discussion—which can take a significant amount of time.

Likewise, researchers must consider how much time, outside of project work, they are willing and able to dedicate to involvement with the community. The research staff must keep the commitment to personally "give back" to the community as a high priority. Since this relationship-building phase must take place well in advance of the start of project planning, it is generally outside the realm of project funding. Most often, researchers volunteer or donate their time to community organizations in order to build rapport, trust, and a sense of commitment to the well-being of the community and its members.

Researcher Reflection

How can a researcher build trust within a funding agency's tight timetable?

Step back and be willing to go slowly and build credibility. And that's difficult because your funding agency usually has a very different timeline. They have a set of things they want to have done in a very limited period of time. You often end up butting heads with project officers about time when the reality is if you want to work with a community, you have to be willing to take the time and build the relationships with the front end and build a sense that you are a person who can be trusted.

(continued)

If you just blast into a community, with your outside timeline, you are not going to get anywhere. So you have to be willing to go slow, even though it does create problems in the immediate sense. But in the long term sense, it is the only way, I think, you can survive and do a good job.

Excerpted from a video interview with Gloria Eldridge, Ph.D., Associate Professor of Psychology, University of Alaska Anchorage

Case Study 2.1

A partnership of local mental health professionals approached researchers at a nearby university expressing a strong interest in studying the prevalence of adolescent depression in their community. The community group conveyed a strong desire to take the lead role in developing a survey instrument for the project (including how it would be administered), determining effective, appropriate participant recruitment strategies, interpreting survey results, and applying results to local mental healthcare services delivery. While the community partners understood that their strength was based in a strong knowledge of community needs and perspectives, they also recognized that the university researchers had the technical and scientific expertise to conduct a rigorous and reliable study. Therefore, the community partners elected not to be involved in data entry or data analysis of survey results.

Given the differing demands of time and technical expertise required for the broad scope of project-related tasks, differing levels of involvement may be appropriate for different partners (Minkler and Wallerstein 2003, p 63). A core principle of community-based participatory research (CBPR) is that all partners are equally involved in all phases of the research process. In reality, since each community is unique in its context, resources, membership, and culture, it is important for individual partnerships to collaboratively determine the role and responsibilities of each partner. It is critical that these decisions are made collaboratively and respectfully, with full acknowledgment and support of community resources as well as the recognition of the burden that the research work might put on community partners. It is also important to recognize and respect the difference between community partners who wish to take on roles that fit their expertise, and when they are looking to learn new skills to enhance capacity.

- What is the overarching importance of community participation?
- How can you ensure that each partner's unique strengths and talents are recognized and encouraged?
- How can scientific rigor be protected and ensured when community partners express a desire to take the lead in certain aspects of the work?
- How can you find ways to transfer new skills to community partners in order to increase their capacity to continue community change after the work of the research is finished?

Case Study 2.2

A funding opportunity was announced that would support work in communities with certain well-defined characteristics. A university research team that reviewed the funding announcement knew of a community that would meet funding criteria and decided to examine the community's problematic issues and strengths in preparation for a possible response to the funding agency. Community concerns that were examined included substance-related interpersonal violence and impoverished neighborhoods. Strengths that emerged included close family relationships, an active community church, and committed community leaders. After identifying strengths and concerns within the community, the research team contacted community leaders about the possibility of a research study in the community. The research team and community leaders agreed that the opportunity could be beneficial to the community in that it may assist the community leaders in their attempts to reduce interpersonal violence and substance abuse. Despite this common ground, the research team and the community leaders had contrasting views of how "community" should be defined, how results derived from the project would be presented, what the roles of community participants would be, and who would fill those roles. Further, the community leaders questioned the long-term commitment of the research team to the community. These disagreements led to several heated exchanges between the research team and the community leaders, and the research team began to question their community choice. However, the research team remained convinced that the proposed project presented a great opportunity for the team and the community. Given this conviction, the research team decided to reaffirm their commitment to the community and to work with the community leaders to move forward with the project. In so doing, the research team looked objectively at needs they had identified as meaningful to the community and attempted to set aside preconceived notions about the community's social issues. Further, the research team took time out to ask the community leaders for support in better understanding how to engage community members at large in program planning and grant writing.

- How can researchers help convey that they are committed to the community and community participants?
- How can researchers work with community leaders to identify common definitions of issues in question, starting with definitions of the community all the way to definitions of what constitutes a strength or weakness?
- How can researchers work with communities to ensure that results of a project are beneficial to the community and its residents before even beginning to collect data?
- What are effective ways for researchers to incorporate community leaders in the planning and design process of a study or grant proposal?

Case Study 2.3

Current published literature prompted researchers' interest in strengths and challenges of African-American grandparents raising grandchildren. Having little experience with members of the local African-American community, the university research team questioned whether they would be accepted by this population, and if they would be trusted enough to play a role in helping study a personal, often sensitive topic. Researchers were able to enter the community by enlisting the support of a liaison—an older colleague who had established deep roots in the local African-American community.

By enlisting her cultural expertise and guidance, the team was able to meet with leaders of two prominent African-American community-based organizations (CBOs) to ask whether the proposed issue was indeed of concern to the local community, and whether the outside research team might play a role helping to study it. Researchers received an enthusiastic response from both groups. They prepared a grant proposal for funds that would be shared with these two local CBOs. The CBOs in turn were instrumental in putting together a strong community advisory board (CAB), assembling individuals to represent the diversity of the community. The CAB's input into phrasing the interview questions, sampling considerations, discussions about the findings, returning findings to the community, and implementing the results back into the community greatly enhanced the quality of the research process, as well as the culturally appropriate interpretation of the findings and of their application in the community. This experience demonstrates how a topic that originates with the interests of outside researchers can, nevertheless, become an issue that is "owned" by the community.

- What are the goals of the research relationship? Are they driven by researcher goals, community goals, or both?
- How do you address sensitive cultural topics with community members?
- How can you create a safe environment for all partners to voice biases, prejudices, and cultural assumptions that might exist?
- What strategies can you put in place to ensure equity among partners, and mutual respect throughout all decision-making processes?
- What issues are involved in data ownership, intellectual property, and dissemination of results?
- When you enter a community via a liaison, how can you ensure an accurate scope of community representation?

Chapter 3
Beginning Partnerships with Communities

Upon completion of **Chapter 3: Beginning Partnerships with Communities**, the reader will be able to:

- Explain the activities necessary to initiate a CBPR project.
- Recognize the importance of community input in effectively planning and carrying out an appropriate participatory research study.

Introduction

The first salient step in CBPR is to find ways to enter a community respectfully. It is important to keep in mind that just as each community is unique, so too are the methods, strategies, and timing required for outside researchers to introduce themselves to the community's members. No one can enter any situation *tabula rasa*; therefore, researchers must be open to differences in values, behaviors, customs, and social and power structures that are unique to the community. Researchers must be careful not to impose *their* definition of community on the group with which they hope to work. They need to use every resource available to develop an informed understanding of the community's realities.

The research team must look at historical records, study current published literature, and engage in experiential learning about the community of interest. Experiential learning involves strategies such as observation, community volunteerism, and conducting interviews

L.W. Roberts, *Community-Based Participatory Research for Improved Mental Healthcare*, DOI 10.1007/978-1-4614-5517-2_3, © Springer Science+Business Media New York 2013 and informational surveys. Researchers should be prepared to let go of their academic or institutional calendars and be willing to work with the timing and pace of the community. For example, strict adherence to an academic calendar may present significant difficulties when working with the seasonal responsibilities of a Midwestern agricultural community.

The cultural values and norms of each individual community must drive both the research process and the creation of a community solution. CBPR must flow according to the timing and pace of the community.

Steven Adelsheim, M.D.,
Professor of Psychiatry, Pediatrics, and Family/Community Medicine, University of New Mexico School of Medicine

---

Chapter 3 focuses on the steps that are required to enter a community and engage its members. Because of the complexity and importance of this partnership-building phase, this chapter is the longest in the book. It explores ways to build credibility for research and form a reciprocal relationship with the community. It also discusses methods of ensuring appropriate representation of the community in the conduct and decision-making aspects of the project.

Researcher Reflection

What's the value of a community being involved on the front end?

A key piece with the community based participatory research is to actively be engaged with the community to the point where they feel comfortable coming to you saying, "We have this question—can you help us?" If they're to the point to where they can raise the question themselves and say we want to do this, then they can start looking for research funding and support on their own.

Excerpted from a video interview with Carl M. Hild, Ph.D., M.S., Assistant Director, Institute for Circumpolar Health Studies, University of Alaska Anchorage

Who Are the Key Leaders and Natural Wise Persons with Whom Trustworthiness and Integrity Must Be Demonstrated?

As outside researchers prepare to enter a community, it is crucial to gain a working knowledge of the community's structures and its systems of power and influence. Such an understanding is best based on the unique circumstances of the community of interest, not on a preconceived or conventional general understanding of a similarly defined group. Researchers must enter a community with full knowledge of the principles of participatory research. They must focus on identifying the community members and resources that will be most helpful in establishing a successful research partnership.

> *When working in the community, the academic researcher is the student, and the community is the teacher. To presume the reverse will prove to be not only false but also fruitless.*
>
> Daryn Reicherter, M.D.,
> Clinical Associate Professor, Department of Psychiatry and Behavioral Sciences, Stanford University

Thoughtful entry into a community begins with the identification of key community individuals and groups who can:

- Assist with networking within the community
- Lend support
- Share insights about the existing hierarchies, power structures, and social networks
- Advocate for the research team and its beneficence
- Communicate the importance and value of research to the greater community

Researchers generally benefit from interacting with as many people as possible early in the relationship-forming process. When researchers rely too heavily on early, limited contacts with few community members, they may proceed with the study basing critical decisions on information that is inaccurate or that presents very limited, unbalanced, or subjective views of the community.

Example:

Local researchers were approached by an enthusiastic Latino community member looking to investigate a community health issue. The university group was confident that having this research partner was a good way to build rapport with the community and to get community perspective in their work. In time it became apparent that the partners had very different research perspectives, creating conflict and disagreement. Also, it became clear that the community partner was not well-liked or trusted by the community, and that he had a reputation for being affiliated with groups that had very clear, very specific agendas. It is critical to determine whether community partners are open to collaboration, or if they bring with them preconceived agendas and divisiveness.

Identifying and engaging individuals with strong voices who are perceived as representative and legitimate by the rest of the community are important early steps in the CBPR process. Researchers are often initially viewed as outsiders, and may only be invited into a community if they are aligned with those who have roles of positive influence in the larger community. The benefits of identifying the "right" individuals in a community to help pave the way for participatory research cannot be overestimated; the outcome of this effort is one of the quickest roads to success or failure.

In many cases, identification of respected or powerful individuals may be difficult, as is gaining a realistic understanding of the extent to which their power truly influences and represents the community. The following examples help illuminate this point.

Examples of Powerful and Influential Individuals

- In many small towns, long-standing residents—those who have resided in the community most of their lives, or members of families with a history in the community for many generations—are highly respected by other residents. These community members, however, might not be treated with similar respect by outsiders who have little knowledge of community history or understanding the social structure.
- An influential leader in a Native community may be a person with strong spiritual and/or cultural values who has earned the respect of community members. These individuals may not *seek* leadership but, rather, are persons elevated to leadership by the community because they are perceived by the community

as having knowledge, wisdom, and skills, and are highly respected by its members (Oldaker).

- In more hidden communities, such as groups of injection drug users, identifying power structures can be difficult. Power is often based on social network position within the community. Observing information patterns or identifying how members are connected sheds important light on the role individuals hold within the network, the connections between individuals in the group, and the position of each individual within the group's social context (Schensul et al. 1999).
- In Amish communities it is age, not youth, that is respected. Amish bishops, preachers, and deacons are chosen by the congregations using a lot system. Positions in the Amish community are held for life.

Sources of Information

The first step in identifying key individuals is the gathering of background information about a community. The research team needs to learn as much as possible about community life and underlying structures to begin open, meaningful communications. For example, important information can be obtained through the following methods.

Methods of Studying a Community's Background

- Archival and library research
- Historical investigation using documents and personal history
- Local narratives and stories
- In vivo observation, perhaps through volunteerism
- Questionnaires or interviews

The information obtained from these and other sources must be gathered, synthesized, and used to inform each step in the relationship-forming process. When reaching out to community members to find answers about structures of power and influence, researchers may find that participants have difficulty answering these questions and may even give contradictory answers. In a geographically defined community, some residents will identify local organizations as important community representatives. They may point to groups such as parent–teacher associations and women's organizations or groups at local religious institutions as the true representatives of the community, as memberships for such groups most often come directly from the community. Other residents, however, may view such organizations as overly concerned with their own agendas, which may take precedence over the good of the community-at-large.

Gathering as much input as possible from community members regarding their perceptions of social structure and systems of power is crucial. This information needs to be carefully evaluated before research teams can arrive at the most accurate picture of where power lies, and how authority and respect influence community life.

Working with Community-Based Organizations

If researchers choose to reach out to community-based organizations (CBOs), it is important to keep in mind that some communities may not be open to new ideas or to partnering with researchers; they may be resistant to change. Researchers may encounter conflicts between community members and individuals affiliated with a community organization. Even within community organizations, group perspective may be divided on an issue based on differences in overall philosophy, values, priorities, assumptions, decision-making, and/or problem-solving styles. Differences among groups can also be based on gender, age, class, race, or sexual orientation. For example, community organizations run mostly by male-dominated groups may have difficulty accepting women as equal partners, or members of a CBO in which a racial hierarchy exists may be unwilling to work with people that have historically been considered more powerful or powerless. While it is true that individual differences can result in conflict and divisiveness on a research team, researchers should first try to understand the mission and goals of the CBO or community group, and determine how they might affect the research project. Groups and organizations that are not open to change or to the vision of the project may actively resist or may generate support to resist any attempts to work toward community change.

Demonstrating thorough knowledge of a community's current situation and relevant history will help present the research team as an informed and sincere potential research partner. It is important that researchers enter organizations well informed about the community's background, but without assuming that they already understand the community. This approach shows the CBO that the researchers have done their homework, and that there is still much to learn about the day-to-day realities of the community. In other words, from the very beginning, the research team continually looks to the community as resident experts whose input is crucial in every step of the process.

Working with Grassroots Activists

Another group that might be a valuable resource to researchers is that of the community's grassroots activists. These are individuals who hold community needs in highest regard and take action on behalf of the community—but do so without clear organizational ties. Unlike "official" community representatives, grassroots group members are not constrained by organizational agendas. Researchers should keep in mind that these individuals often have a history of advocating and taking action on behalf of community needs. Such advocacy and action may support the potential research team if perceptions of the community's needs happen to align. On the other hand, if the activists do not see the research agenda as legitimate or beneficial for the community, they may become a barrier to the study. Thorough information-gathering early in the process will provide researchers with information about the grassroots community groups, and whether the fundamental priorities of these groups align with the goals of the project.

Multiple Sources of Power and Influence

One challenge that may arise within a community is the presence of multiple sources of power and influence that are at odds with each other. This may result in a situation where a too-close alliance or partnership with one source may alienate another—resulting in the research collaboration being conflicted before it begins. Ideally, the solution would be to find common ground between the opposing community powers and offer ways to engage them in a single partnership that everyone can support. If such a joint position is achieved, the researchers will have made a significant contribution to the community already. However, if reaching unity in purpose is not possible, the researchers may need to evaluate carefully whether or not to pursue research work with that particular community.

To summarize, there are many sources of leadership and many forms of community representation. The research team must take utmost care to contact all potential sources of power and respect, and involve each in the research planning process. Only on rare occasions does a community have just one easily identifiable leader through whom the team will work exclusively. Often, a significant early challenge of CBPR is recognizing that there are many legitimate voices, all of which need to be heard, valued, and respected.

> If you underestimate the amount of time it takes to build a relationship and develop trust, you will likely face a community suspicious or "put off" by feeling pushed too hard too quickly – the process will be slowed.

When and How Do Researchers Approach a Community?

In addition to ensuring that the research team talks to the "right" people in a community, they must also enter a community at a time that is appropriate and logical from the community's perspective.

Timing Considerations

Entering a community with a specific topic in mind, while that community is struggling with a completely different issue, may lead to failure and perceptions of irrelevance at best, and ill will at worst. For example, if a community is struggling with repeated suicides among its adolescents, it may not welcome researchers who are interested in taking blood samples from children to explore the genetic basis of mathematics disabilities. However, if instead the researchers recognize the community's real struggle and enter with a genuine offer of assistance with suicide prevention, their timing will align with the community's needs.

Example:
Academic researchers joined forces with local organizations to conduct a formative study of community knowledge of Alzheimer's disease, and to assess ways of disseminating information about it in the Latino community. Teams of research staff members interviewed families, service providers, and community groups to identify differences in the cultural meaning of Alzheimer's disease, and potential distribution channels for disseminating information on diagnosis, care, and management of the disease. Researchers found that families were troubled by the term "Alzheimer's disease" because it was associated with the loss of control and mental health difficulties. This might have resulted in the community's reluctance to participate in the study. Therefore, researchers decided to identify themselves to families as people investigating health problems associated with aging. They planned to discuss symptoms first, and only later discuss dementias.

The timing for starting a research project must also take into consideration whether a community will be able to accommodate the full scope of work. While establishing a specific project schedule is difficult early in the CBPR process, researchers must generally determine if a community is in a position to provide the hours, months, and possibly years that will likely be required to complete the research. Some CBPR studies are completed within 12 months' time. Others can take 3 years or more. Knowing what level of commitment people can make is important before engaging them in a process that might not be completed, resulting in community dissatisfaction and researcher frustration.

Entering a Community Respectfully

In addition to appropriate timing, researchers must enter the community in a respectful manner. Most importantly, to promote concepts of respect, collaboration, and partnership (the cornerstones of participatory research), they must dedicate appropriate time and attention to mutual trust-building with the target community. Developing mutual trust is a multifaceted process that will lead to the cyclical information-sharing and feedback that is crucial to the CBPR process. Over time, this mutual trust will shape the nature of the interactions between the research team and the community. Also, these ongoing interactions will determine the degree of collaboration, cooperation, and respect that develops among the members of the partnership. Because of the cyclical nature of this trust-building process, it can be time-intensive but cannot be skipped or shortened.

Methods for Building Trust

There are a number of effective methods for building trust among members of the research partnership. Many of the following may prove helpful as researchers begin to engage with a community, as well as during the later stages of the research process. Although these approaches are presented separately, they are intimately tied to one another and often co-occur in ongoing fashion throughout a research study.

Trust-Building Approaches

- *Building Trust through Existing Linkages.* The trust-building process is greatly enhanced when outside researchers have the support of existing relationships with individuals, groups, and/or organizations within the target community—such as mental healthcare providers, coalitions, and health service organizations. These existing linkages can send a message to the community-at-large that the research team is trustworthy, which may help overcome prejudices that exist. They also provide valuable connections to assist researchers in sharing information about the potential research partnership, conducting community education efforts, and establishing the research team's commitment to "give back" to the community.
- *Building Trust through New Relationships with Individuals and Groups.* When researchers do not have existing relationships, they must find ways to become personally involved with community members in their natural environment. Partnering with community members for CBPR purposes always requires a certain level of personal involvement, which can be forged at both an individual and group level.

  Creating connections with individual community members can often be best accomplished by entering through group interactions. Participating in a group event, such as serving as a featured speaker on a topic relevant to the proposed research, may help members of the community see the research team as a legitimate source of information and support. When a research team chooses to develop personal relationships at the group level, it is important to keep in mind that communities differ vastly with regard to levels of helplessness and dependency, capacity and resources, and openness or closedness. Personal styles of interaction with groups (and individuals, for that matter) must be adapted to these factors of community functioning.

Given this context, entering a community is always a social movement. Whenever groups begin to organize, the need for members to understand more about each other emerges, as well as the need to understand the personal situations of other members of the group. Entry into a community by the research team is therefore a reciprocal social exchange. During these early attempts at community entry, researchers should begin the process of ongoing self-reflection and building on the new knowledge gained from their new CBPR partners. The research team must allow the community to set the pace and the timing for this relationship and trust-building, and not impose an external timeline onto the process. The most important feature of this entry is to become recognized as a legitimate and important part of a group with something of value to offer for the good of the greater community. Being personable, open, respectful, kind, and flexible are requirements. Groups and individuals need to feel that they are heard and understood and that they are taken seriously and approached as equals. They must not feel patronized, lectured to, or taken for granted.

In addition, researchers should collaborate with individuals or groups that have a strong community presence. These relationships will provide a valuable asset for organizing a research project. Such community partners can help generate interest and attendance when process matters are discussed or information is presented to the community-at-large (which is discussed in later chapters).

- *Building Trust by Accumulating Relevant Knowledge about a Given Community.* The process of building trust at group and individual levels is often best facilitated by researchers gaining as much knowledge as possible about the community, with the clear understanding that such knowledge is often an outsider's view and needs to be supplemented by more subjective, personal perspectives of the community's members. Bringing a context of knowledge is important, even if it must be tempered and contextualized. Several areas of information are necessary including, most simply, information about the community background and culture.

Community background. Outside researchers need to be proactive in information-gathering to gain a clear understanding of community history. They must learn everything they can about the community and its members. This can be accomplished through reviewing available records, direct observation, interviews, and participating in community life. Researchers need to find effective, creative ways to engage individuals and groups operating at different levels in order to gain a more complete picture of community history, experience, and context. Such work is often helpful later in the CBPR process, when researchers may wish to use information about individual members to identify key people who can fill the research roles as community experts.

Community culture. Perhaps even more importantly, outside researchers need to be proactive in gathering information about community culture. It is vital to have an understanding of the community's cultural norms so that outsiders (such as the research team) can understand what is expected of them, start to break down cultural barriers, and begin to gain respect from the community. In some communities outside researchers are perceived as having superior or privileged status, a perception that can adversely affect relationship-building. In others, people may be hesitant because they hold stereotypes about researchers as intrusive, self-serving, unhelpful, and removed. Addressing these issues early on is crucial to communicating the concept of equal partnership to community members. It is also important for the research team to remember that during all interactions with the community, they are being watched and evaluated by its members. First impressions can literally make or break the success of a CBPR effort.

- *Building Trust through Listening to and Observing the Obvious and the Subtle.* Outside researchers are best served by first approaching the community as simple listeners and observers, and engaging in community life in a nonintrusive and non-overbearing manner. The ideal way to get to know a community is to experience it firsthand. Finding but not forcing opportunities for interaction, not necessarily focused on research, is an excellent way of making the research team members known to a community and to begin to form personal relationships. Sometimes watching a community basketball game may be time very well spent; or volunteering to help with a community clean-up effort can demonstrate enormous goodwill.

During informal interactions with the community, researchers still need to keep in mind that first impressions may be misleading. When interacting with a new person (i.e., the researcher), community members may put their best foot forward, responding to questions with answers they believe are expected or that hide some community realities they may not want an outsider to know. This is true, perhaps especially, in the context of early research interactions (such as during data-gathering on key individuals or community needs vis-a-vis research topics). It is important for outside researchers to be aware that a community's or community member's initial responses may not accurately represent individual or collective realities. It may not be until some trust has been established that researchers can begin to rely fully on the information that is shared. Appropriate, respectful trust-building is required to create community–researcher partnerships that are honest and equitable.

- *Building Trust through Sharing Information.* As is inherent in any relationship built on trust and respect, all people involved in the partnership need to share information. That is, the flow of information needs to be multidirectional and cannot always simply be from the community to the researcher. At times it may be valuable for the researchers to share information regarding their personal, family, community, and cultural realities—a sharing that may help break down barriers between the community and the research team. Although this may prove challenging to researchers who have been trained to maintain firm boundaries between the researcher and the researched, it is often imperative to do so to achieve information-sharing goals.

That said, researchers must remain true to their own values and beliefs. They need to find a balance that meets both the need for trust-building and the need for being true to themselves. Once researchers find a balance, they must consistently work to maintain that balance throughout the work of the study. Building the research relationship on a foundation of sharing creates a partnership based on interconnectedness between people, which may blur the line between researcher and community member, while strengthening the concept of equity, mutual respect, and partnership.

Information-sharing does not just stop there. It also involves shared discussion of the research topic, design, and outcome.

This process is so central to CBPR that it is discussed in multiple additional contexts in this chapter and chapters to follow.

It's important to "really listen to" and "really see" the people you hope to work with. Closely observe facial expressions, and tone and pitch of voice in addition to what is being said. Recognize that silence can be an active communication tool; what is not said may be as important as what is. Also, realize that small gestures such as smiling and shaking hands might be speaking volumes to your potential community partners.

- *Building Trust through Invited Collaborations and Cooperation.* While most CBPR researchers struggle to introduce themselves into a new target community, some communities actually initiate the relationship by reaching out to research teams for consultation or to conduct a study on specific community needs. The CBPR research team is held accountable to the community and is expected to consider its input every step of the way. This type of partnership tends to be most common among rural or frontier community health agencies that are generally too overburdened to engage in research on their own.

Outside research teams may also be brought in on collaborative research projects initiated by communities. In this type of relationship, the research team supplies technical scientific expertise, and community leaders contribute their expert knowledge of local needs and perspectives. Joint responsibility for specific aspects of the project requires a united approach in which all partners make important contributions to the project. The details of this united effort must be defined in depth and understood at the outset, and committed to by both the researchers and the community. This type of CBPR model serves to lessen the fears of community members who believe that outside researchers conducting a study may inadvertently disempower a community and take over control. Creating a detailed research agreement early on also helps to prevent a situation in which researchers may become subservient by giving up too much control to the community, and seriously affecting the scientific integrity of the study.

Even in situations in which the research team's involvement is solicited by a community or an organization within a community, the research team needs to talk to its members, collect relevant statistics and other information, and conduct the preliminary work necessary to demonstrate that a) the project's topic is of importance to the community, and b) CBPR principles are being applied. Also, the research team and the community partners need to co-present early study information to the community, with confidence that the project will attract widespread community support that goes beyond the group of individuals that originally solicited the researchers.

Final Notes About When and How to Enter Communities

The initial organizational phase of a CBPR project can take a considerable amount of time; just how much time will be unique to each project and determined by the characteristics and context of the community. If the research team is not trained and practiced in cyclical and self-reflective strategies, this first crucial step in the CBPR process may result in failure. That is, the community may decide not to participate in the project and to not grant entry to the researchers. It is not at all uncommon for this initial project phase to last as long as 6–12 months. There are no shortcuts and there are no exceptions.

Taking adequate time to build a strong relationship with the community, in the end, is time very well spent. Since this phase of CBPR takes a considerable amount of time, it is best to form community relationships well in advance of starting a research project. That way, when researchers are looking for project funding, they can demonstrate their capacity to carry out CBPR by demonstrating the existence of solid community ties. Having a strong link to the community already in place can help demonstrate the credibility of community partners, as well as ways in which researchers are aware of issues that are important to the community, and of potential barriers to the project or to community participation. Establishing the cooperation of the community also ensures that important elements of the project (work plan, schedule, budget, etc.) have been determined with community input.

It is important to note that the reluctance of some communities to participate in research often has distant roots in past experiences with researchers who were less than respectful in how they entered and exited the community. Researchers attempting to enter a community must have knowledge of its previous research encounters. Research team members must demonstrate that they are aware of the past wrongdoings and will do everything in their power to avoid repeating them. This will be discussed further in future chapters.

Researcher Reflection

How do you build on relationships that are already established?

I think that the first strategy we do try to use is do we have anybody on our team or on our staff who already has a personal relationship with that group and use that as the bridge. Then, slowly, as the project is being developed and implemented, then the actual research team can begin to develop a relationship with those people as well. So we tag-team it initially if that's the best way to enter the community and start building trust and a sense of cooperation.

Excerpted from a video interview with Karen Ward, Ph.D., Professor and Director, Center for Human Development, University of Alaska Anchorage

What Information Is Appropriate to Share About the Scientific Questions, the Methodology, and the Anticipated Risks and Benefits to the Community and to Individual Participants?

In keeping with the principles of participatory research, ongoing information-sharing between the research team and community partners is essential to the success of the study. One of the main benefits of the CBPR process is the co-learning that occurs from ongoing information-sharing between partners. Also, through ongoing discussion each member of the partnership is able to voice individual ideas, perspectives, or concerns about any aspect of the process.

Given the commitment to this process, participatory research is, by nature and definition, highly ethical, thereby minimizing risk and increasing benefit to the community. By involving community partners in every aspect of the study process, from developing the research question to disseminating results, participatory research embraces the cornerstones of ethically responsible research as its highest priority.

Specifically, CBPR upholds all of the following ethics principles.

- Respect for persons
- Non-maleficence (to do no harm)
- Beneficence (to do good)
- Justice (fairness and equity)
- Veracity (truth-telling)

All discussions and decision-making involving research partners must be conducted and recorded at a literacy and competency level that is appropriate to all. Also, a commitment to ethics must be agreed to by all partners in considering the impact on the community at large in all decisions regarding the CBPR project.

As reflected in participatory research principles, all elements of the research process must be discussed and decided upon by all parties who hold positions of power and decision-making within the partnership. Minimally, adherence to ethical and community-respectful practices implies that the research partnership collaborates on and clearly spells out all of the following issues (Adams et al. 2004; NAPCRG 1998).

Information-Sharing Requirements

1. Clarification of roles and responsibilities of all collaborators, from research leaders to community volunteers
2. Terms of and agreements underlying all aspects of the partnership
3. Clarification of all issues surrounding confidentiality
4. Procedures for incorporation of new collaborators
5. Specification of methods for resolving disagreements or conflicts
6. Negotiation of all research goals and objectives
7. Formulation of the research question
8. Specification of the project's methods
9. Specification of the project's duration
10. Discussion of analytic strategies and plans
11. Clarification of data control issues (strategies for collection, storage, and use of data)
12. Statement of the desired outcomes of the research and plans for implementation of findings into the community, if appropriate
13. Plans for dissemination of results

While these requirements uphold the principles of CBPR in its strictest sense, there may be instances, particularly in well-organized communities, when authority and power occasionally change hands rather than remaining equal. Communities that are especially well organized may be equipped to conduct their own research, but may not have the resources to take the time from day-to-day community obligations. With less-organized communities, organizing the group may well become part of the CBPR process in order to create a starting point from which to formulate the research plan. Other communities present a mixed bag of organization and capacity. As has been stated earlier in this book and will be stated again—each community presents its own set of strengths, needs, and resources. Each CBPR project will consist of a unique set of guidelines and agreements dictating process and responsibilities, lending even more support to the importance of joining the community in advance of the start of the study, and learning everything possible about day-to-day community life.

Information-sharing involves as many community members as feasible and begins with the foundations of research (clear communication of items 1–5 above), continues with the negotiation and sharing of the research question (items 6–7 above), moves to the formulation of the research process (items 8–11 above), and ends with the shared vision of outcomes dissemination (items 12–13 above).

For example, once the research question is formulated, the researchers can present to the partners the process options to consider that lie within the available personnel and other resources of the community. The researchers then explain their logic, efficacy, and limitations. This aspect of a participatory study serves to demystify research methodology and puts decisions about the process in the hands of the people so that, early on, collaboration in decision-making becomes a tool of empowerment.

Involving all partners in each aspect of the research endeavor is required for the project to be truly participatory. It is important to note that a lack of formal education never disqualifies community members from inclusion in this process. Participatory research centers on a collaborative effort, where everyone knows some things, but no one knows everything. Working together, all partners will know more about each other, and about different *ways* of knowing. Working side by side with community partners every step of the way strengthens the cultural validity of the results, minimizes harm, supports community education and autonomy, increases mutual learning, values diverse perspectives, and will likely result in positive community change.

Community Member Reflection

What is most important to the community members who participate?

I felt like by participating we were contributing to improving services for children and families. Then there's this feeling of, somebody respects my opinion as a parent enough that they want to collect this information, that you're not just a mere parent of a kid that has special needs. But, there's added things that you've learned through that experience of raising this child that are going to benefit other people and somebody wants to capture that. I think that's great! Some of us have really had to go through a lot to get to the point where our kids are successful and as independent as they are at this point. And we like to share that information. It's also good to be able to tell people what isn't working in systems and the challenges and the grief that families deal with. That's not always something that happens or is included or considered as part of the plan for what researchers expect to get out of it, but they probably should be aware that going through these kinds of survey tools and being asked questions about your family resiliency and what is or isn't working. It does stir up some of those grief and sadness issues for us because it does ask us to compare where our kids are compared to other people's children. And once again we see that they're not keeping up.

Excerpted from a video interview with Cheryl Scott, Parent Navigator Training Coordinator, Anchorage, Alaska

Community members involved in CBPR reported feelings of excitement and hope during first meetings with the research team. *"For the first time ever, someone who could really help was asking us about our needs, and we were going to do whatever it took to do it right, even if that meant some disagreement or frustration along the way. We felt so strong and hopeful, and we knew our community would someday be better for going through this."*

How Do Researchers Figure Out Ways to Minimize Risk to the Community?

Historical wrongdoing in research involving human participants has resulted in federal regulations and guidelines designed to reduce the risk of future harm. Although these standards protect *individual* research participants, nothing is currently in place to protect *communities* from harm. It is the responsibility of the research team to discuss protection guidelines early on, and to affirm that one of the study's top priorities is to be watchful for potential risks to the community.

To safeguard against risk to groups involved in participatory research, the concepts of beneficence, justice, veracity, and autonomy that protect individuals should be applied as community protections as well.

Questions to Ask When Developing Community Safeguards

- When does a group require separate ethical considerations not included in individual safeguard guidelines and requirements?
- How should informed consent guidelines be modified to take into account particular group characteristics?
- What new privacy considerations exist in a community when members (research partners and participants) know each other very well?
- How do close-knit social networks create difficulty maintaining privacy of participants?
- How does the researcher deal with differing opinions of group representatives from one community when making decisions that affect all?
- How can the problem of community stigmatization from research results be addressed?
- How should questions of ownership of data and results be addressed?
- How are individual rights protected when the community owns that data?
- What confidentiality considerations arise when community partners are involved in all aspects of the study?

These and other difficult issues should be discussed and decisions about procedures to minimize research risks should be agreed upon by all partners. Once the requirements for community protections have been developed, the next struggle may come in trying to put them into practice.

Recommendations for Reducing Risk

- IRBs overseeing the research must contain members who are knowledgeable about CBPR.
- IRB membership overseeing the research should include representatives with CBPR experience.
- There must be acknowledgement that community partners often act as informal IRBs with their own culturally and situationally influenced standards.

In community-based research, it is crucial that information regarding the study be made available to community members in language that is understandable to all, particularly information about participant protections and rights. Anyone who is involved or simply interested in the research project must be able to fully understand every aspect of the study to make an informed decision about whether to participate.

It must be made absolutely clear that even though individuals agree to participate in the study, they have the right to withdraw at any time without repercussions or judgment. Given the centrality of ethical conduct in research for CBPR, a separate and detailed discussion of ethical safeguards is presented in Chapter 4.

Confidentiality and Anonymity

In community research, protecting confidentiality and anonymity of the community and its members may become an area of concern. Will community members feel free to disclose personal information to research team members who also reside in the community? How will daily community life be affected among individuals holding different roles in the research process? How will relationships change between those involved in the research and those who have elected not to participate?

> Change is a journey of the many steps it takes for a community
> to move from one place to another. Responsibility for commu-
> nity change is shared by all the people who work together, each
> step of the way, to make change happen – they have provided
> leadership.

How Are Community Advisory Boards Developed, and How Will Healthy, Effective Functioning Be Facilitated?

The success of any CBPR project is greatly enhanced by establishing a community advisory board (CAB). The importance and possible benefits of the CAB cannot be overstated; therefore, this section of Chapter 3 provides detailed information on how to establish and maintain this essential advisory component.

The research team, which includes researchers and community leaders, generally initiates the process of forming a CAB for the project. Comprising a group of diverse community representatives, the CAB's primary purpose is to serve as a liaison between the researchers and the community-at-large.

The CAB helps to ensure that the voice of the community is heard in all aspects of the research, giving community partners a sense of ownership in both the process and the product. As such, it is vital that CAB membership represents the full scope of community opinions, cultures, and values. Not only does the CAB assist in the day-to-day details of running a CBPR project, it advocates for community rights and facilitates disclosure of information about the research project to the community. CAB members must be fully informed and involved vis-a-vis research procedures, and need to have an appreciation of the larger purposes of the CBPR project.

Selection and Coordination of CAB Members

In establishing a board that will truly inform the research process from the perspective of the community, the research team must give careful thought to accurate and thorough representation. It is helpful to include a blend of community members, activists, and leaders—all of whom work collaboratively and supportively with the research team. The board should represent the diversity of the community as is appropriate. Community diversity may include the following:

- Age
- Gender
- Ethnicity or race
- Professional affiliations and choices (blue collar, white collar, pink collar)
- Educational level
- Religion
- Socioeconomics and income levels
- Special interest groups
- Self-identified cultural groups within the community

When forming a CAB, the research team must pay attention to power differentials that exist in the community. Since a fully representative CAB membership will include different subgroups from within the community, a hierarchy may form among CAB members that reflects existing power differentials. To help ensure smooth group functioning, the research team should strongly emphasize that existing community power structures must not extend to the relationship of CAB members within the context of CAB activities. This philosophy is critical in ensuring that an equitable, democratic process will guide the work of the board.

Ideally, researchers should be trained in group process and conflict resolution, providing them with the skills to promote effective group functioning and cooperation across power structures and other perceived subgroups. Organized, facilitated dialogue about respect and equity of influence among CAB members must take place early on. Although it may be difficult to create equity and respect among CAB members who experience hierarchies and power structures outside of the CBPR project, strategies must be created and employed within the group to demonstrate equity among all members of the research team and CAB. These strategies may include, but are not limited to, conducting role play, providing education about small group behavior, establishing task-oriented processes, and establishing thoughtful meeting protocol.

Prior to agreeing to serve on a board, member candidates must be made aware of the long-term commitment and personal demands inherent in research project involvement. Above all, the research team should resist the common practice of seeking exclusively mental healthcare providers, community leaders, and other prominent community citizens to serve as members. These individuals represent the community's power base only and do not make for a well-balanced and fully representative board.

Example:
The partners of the academic research team were primarily representatives from community-based organizations. Since the study topic focused on teenage drug use, the CAB decided that in order to more accurately represent the community, a parent of a drug-using teen should be included in the CAB membership. The neighbor of a CAB member, whose son had been involved with drugs, was asked to join the CAB to represent the parent perspective.

While this is a viable strategy to broaden the scope of community representation, it is important to note that just as no one group can accurately represent a population, no individual can represent a specific subpopulation. Each member of the CAB may represent a specific faction of the community, but creating opportunities to hear from the larger community must be ongoing.

Involvement of the CAB in the Research Process

Because CAB members come from the community, they can inform the research process about cultural, social, and health issues and value priorities, as well as ensure that a suitable process is in place for conducting respectful, nonexploitative research as perceived by community members. An initial schedule for CAB meeting days/ times should be established early on. The study will benefit by creating a meeting timeline that attends to members' personal and other commitments outside of CAB activities.

Since the CAB serves as a liaison between community members and the research partners, its members' input on all aspect of the study is important.

Advisory Contributions of CAB Members

- Forming the research question
- Writing the project mission statement
- Recruiting research team members from the community

- Developing the research protocol
- Developing useful and appropriate participant recruitment and retention strategies
- Establishing meeting formats for the CAB and the community-at-large
- Reviewing the informed consent form
- Reviewing sampling strategies
- Contributing to data collection procedures, data storage, and perhaps even data analysis
- Contextualizing data collected to support appropriate interpretation
- Reviewing the process for releasing outcome information about data collected
- Discussing the implications of findings
- Participating in strategic planning to translate findings into community action

Some of the following purposes and functions may also be associated with well-developed and cooperative CABs that have strong and positive partnerships with the research team.

Other CAB Contributions

- Ensuring that interventions, assessments, surveys, and other research procedures are appropriate for the community.
- Supplying input into development of materials about the study (e.g., brochures, flyers, consent forms, debriefing sheets) that (a) appropriately and accurately reflect community values and culture, (b) are written in appropriate language(s) and at appropriate reading and comprehension levels, (c) are culturally sensitive, and (d) present adequate information for truly informed consent of community members.
- Serving as a liaison between community members, research participants, and outside researchers, by voicing community concerns or advocating for community rights (Strauss et al. 2001).

> *In the end, the academic researcher and the community-based partner are accountable less to each other and more to the population they serve.*
>
> Daryn Reicherter, M.D.,
> Clinical Associate Professor, Department of Psychiatry and Behavioral Sciences, Stanford University

Community advisory board members provide invaluable input in identifying and prioritizing community needs. This helps ensure that the research methodology is consistent with community characteristics, aligns with community needs, and provides continual feedback during the entire study process. When community members are well represented on an advisory board, the community maintains a strong, consistent, and meaningful voice in the partnership and in the outcomes of the study. A community well represented by a CAB is more likely to develop a sense of ownership and responsibility for the project, investment in translating research findings into action, and willingness to collaborate on future research efforts.

Tips for a Well-Functioning CAB

Although each CAB will offer its own unique strengths and challenges, a few practical suggestions for operating an effective and healthy board are applicable to most, if not all, situations. The following strategies are among those that can be implemented by the research team:

CAB Operating Guidelines

- *Meetings.* The CAB is best served by meeting at a time and place that is convenient for all members. In addition to in-person meetings, the research team can offer options of e-mail, teleconference, and/or web conference formats.

- *Size*. The CAB benefits from maintaining an appropriate group size. The board must be large enough to truly represent the community, but small enough that each voice can be heard and that all members can contribute to the work of the CAB.
- *Purpose*. The CAB will be most successful if the board is active in planning and conducting the work of the study and not simply an advisory group. As members work together on important aspects of the research, cohesion and commitment are strengthened.
- *Conflict*. The CAB will be most helpful to the research team if they understand the cyclical nature of a CAB, including a likely initial "storming period" as members work through process rules, procedure, purpose, etc. Although it may be disconcerting for members to experience conflict early in the process, storming is often necessary for eventual group cohesion.
- *Recognition*. CAB volunteers are taking time out of their everyday lives to contribute to the work of the research team. Thus, the research team needs to find ways to show appreciation and recognition for the CAB's contributions.

Final Comments About CABs

Although forming and maintaining an effective community advisory board require a considerable amount of time and effort on the part of the research team, the CAB is a crucial element that must not be skipped. A healthy CAB provides a forum for researchers and community representatives to discuss the focus, purpose, process, risks, benefits, and impact of the project within an equitable, respectful context. A healthy CAB ensures that a CBPR effort is exactly what it should be: a community-based program that allows for equal participation across all levels of a community within the context of an equal partnership with a well-informed, well-meaning research team. Often the success of a CAB rests on the ability of the research team or the principal researcher to make CAB members feel a true and relevant part of the research process and of a project that serves the well-being of the community. This requires good communication and interpersonal skills on the part of the research team, especially its leaders.

How Should Values Conflicts and Disagreements Be Addressed?

Regardless of how hard a research team works on developing and maintaining a respectful partnership with a community, a time may come when conflicts or arguments arise. When this occurs, differences of opinion are not to be avoided, feared, or viewed as signs of failure. Rather, these challenges are best approached as opportunities to demonstrate that the research team has an attitude of openness, collaborative problem-solving, cooperation, and non-defensiveness. In other words, both the research team and community partners need to learn and recognize that when disagreements do occur, a preexisting safe, respectful environment will help foster creative, positive solutions.

Collaborative Resolution of Conflict

Conflict is a natural part of group formation and collaboration. Disagreements that occur within the group or among partners must be addressed collaboratively, as opposed to using a competitive or hierarchical group management approach. Developing a strong capacity for empathy among the partners will improve and strengthen the group's platform for decision-making, project management, and conflict resolution. Most often, new CBPR partnership groups gain more insight and enhanced problem-solving skills as time goes on. As group members improve their interpersonal and communication skills, they become excellent role models for the larger community.

As the partnership develops, new members may be added who possess differing theoretical, methodological, or experiential skills from others in the group. When this occurs, the potential for conflict may be reintroduced. Given the dynamic nature of group processes and of the participatory process, reoccurring issues regarding the roles of the partners, intended process, or outcome of the research project may need to be addressed. The potential for conflict during the partnership should be acknowledged, and even anticipated, by building in mechanisms for its resolution.

Seeking Outside Help to Resolve Conflict

Occasionally, conflict and disagreement may reach proportions that feel unmanageable, and assistance from a skilled facilitator may be required. Just as with any conflict situation, such an occurrence does not reflect a failure but instead represents an opportunity. Discussions with a skilled facilitator will inevitably lead to new understandings and skills among the partners and will serve to expand the group's empathic, interpersonal, and communication skills.

If a facilitator is brought in, all discussions that take place around the points of conflict or disagreement must include appropriate representation of all diverging views. Plenty of time must be allocated to hear all opinions and to ensure that input from all individuals who wish to participate is heard and valued. If the discussions are kept brief or include only select community leaders or stakeholders, the greater community will likely question the legitimacy of the process and its decisions, since clearly all perspectives are not equally and carefully considered.

If needed, facilitated discussions may take place on a number of occasions with different community members to get a broad range of perspectives and to be certain that all sides of the story are heard. Some communities may be deeply divided over mental health issues. Often segments of marginalized or vulnerable populations represent a collective viewpoint that is in contrast to the larger community position. Failure to hear a broad representation of perspectives will likely lead to the exclusion of the voice of a particular group that is vital to the project and resulting community change.

Withdrawal of Partners or Project Termination Due to Conflict

Occasionally, a partner may choose to withdraw, a community may decide to discontinue a project, or research may be stopped for other reasons. It is important to note that a critical, ethical point for all research is the right of the participant to withdraw from the project at any time. This right is also extended in CBPR to the research team and community partners. As noted earlier, ethical agreements are negotiated by the research team and the community (or its representatives) at the *outset* of the project and serve to guide the participatory process throughout. At all points during a CBPR study, ethics need to be the overriding determinant of behaviors and actions for all partners. More information on conflict resolution and partnership termination is included in Chapter 4.

In a balanced partnership, leadership roles may shift back and forth depending on who has the expertise on a particular issue. Full partnership between outside researchers and community representatives takes time to establish and the amount of time required cannot be underestimated. It requires careful development of trust, skills, confidence, knowledge, shared vision, and dynamic interaction of values and perspectives that occurs through ongoing respectful dialogue. Doing so respectfully, planfully, carefully, ethically, and *consistently* is the hallmark of CBPR (Wallerstein 1999; Friere 1970).

Core Principles of Participatory Research

- Research partners actively set the project agenda.
- The research should benefit the community by providing tools to analyze conditions and make informed decisions collectively.
- The relationship between researchers and community members should be collaborative and based on dialogical co-learning.
- The process should develop the capacity of community people to acquire and use knowledge from which they might be normally excluded.
- The process should be democratic, enabling the participation of a wide diversity of people.
- Outcomes should be based primarily on the goals of community partners.

Researcher Reflection

How do you work through conflict and find common ground?

I think the common ground is to go to what the product will be. Because you're in the community you're doing research because there is something that either needs to be: it's a problem, it needs to be fixed, it needs to be made better, it needs to be augmented. If you can bring people together to agree on what things would look like or what they will look like when they're better then you can begin to work back and begin to realize that mostly everything else is a disagreement about how to get to that point. So start with the vision of how this is going to look when it's good and how the community is going to look and what they want and then you go back and try to figure out how to get there.

Excerpted from a video interview with Gloria Eldridge, Ph.D., Associate Professor of Psychology, University of Alaska Anchorage

Case Study 3.1

The academic researchers joined forces with local organizations to conduct a formative study of community knowledge of Alzheimer's disease, and to assess ways of disseminating information about it in the Latino community. Members of the research staff interviewed families, service providers, and community institutions to identify differences in the meaning of Alzheimer's disease, and potential distribution channels for accurate information on diagnosis and management of the disease. Researchers found that families were troubled by the term "Alzheimer's disease" because it was associated with the loss of control and mental health problems, both of which were heavily stigmatized in the community. There was widespread fear that being associated with the study would reflect negatively on families. This likely would have resulted in overall community reluctance to participate in the study. Therefore, researchers decided to identify themselves to families as people investigating health issues associated with aging.

They planned to discuss symptoms first, and only later, after some general education and information-sharing with the community, would the research team discuss dementias.

- How do you locate and engage community partners who can share accurate information about the greater community?
- How do you balance your assumptions about the community with the sameness or diversity that actually exists in the community of focus?
- How do you demonstrate credibility and trustworthiness to different subgroups within the community?
- How can you ensure that the research staff remains open to the situations of everyday community life, without judgment, assumptions, or influence?

Case Study 3.2

A program director within the city government of a community wanted research to be conducted that would enable the city to make changes to public safety programs. The individual contacted a former minister of the community who was working at a consulting firm in another state to initiate a study that would explore behaviors that led to detainment for acute alcohol detoxification. The director of the consulting firm formed a permanent field office in the community headed by a local hospital administrator who was to coordinate the study. An initial planning meeting was held at the public safety office in the community to gather public opinions. After this meeting, the consulting firm subcontracted the study to a national research center that specialized in studies on alcohol abuse. The subcontracted research team formed two distinct planning entities: a steering committee, consisting of local indigenous community leaders, and a technical advisory group, consisting primarily of nonindigenous, nonlocal professionals. The study was to focus on distribution and consumption of alcohol, detention, and cultural changes in the community. Trained staff with expertise in alcohol and culture collected data from a convenience sample of indigenous community members over 15 years of age.

After data collection and analysis were completed under the guidance of the technical advisory group, the findings of the study were disseminated by the group via news releases and public community meetings on the same day. The next morning, the local newspaper's lead story was entitled, Alcohol Destroying Community. Soon after, the story was picked up by the Associated Press and broadcast across the USA, clearly identifying the community. Community leaders and members were surprised by and appalled at the original newspaper article and the national exposure. Subsequently, town hall meetings were held to address concerns and allow for questions about study findings and the process used to disseminate the information.

- How is this scenario an example of poor partnership building?
- In what ways did the researchers try to build collaboration?
- Why was the collaboration that was developed ultimately not successful?
- How could value conflicts and disagreements have been identified and addressed up front?
- How can attempts be made to rebuild relationships with community leaders and members after an action that is perceived by the community as a betrayal of trust?

Case Study 3.3

After attending a conference on child health and abuse prevention a researcher decided to initiate a similar program in her local community. She arranged meetings with the board of directors of the local child protection agency, and with community healthcare leaders. Both groups were enthusiastic about helping with the project. After several meetings, the team was prepared to delegate initial tasks to begin the project. The child protection agency partners had experience with child abuse and protection issues, grant writing, and simple administrative structure. The healthcare group had strengths in medical and health issues, education, and research. Tasks were delegated to each group based on its strengths. The group authored, as its early task, a common mission statement that was to guide all project work, from the initial research to results interpretation and eventual program implementation. All members agreed that it was essential to come together early in project planning to define a common goal. Team members recognized that although there was some group tension early on, and that it was a learning experience for researchers and practitioners to work together, it was critical to remember that everyone was working in the same direction toward their common goal, that they respected each other's strengths, and that each group's work was important in accomplishing all project goals.

Important Issues to Address

- How are community partners selected? What are the expectations and assumptions of each?
- What local issues may complicate the early partnership? Are there hierarchies or power structures that could influence early work?
- To what extent do problems involve an agency view versus a community view?
- What are options to make early partnership-forming activities successful or more efficient?
- How do you determine the strengths of the partners?
- Should all project work involve collaboration or will tasks be divided among partners?

Chapter 4
Finding Common Ground Within the Partnership

Upon completion of **Chapter 4: Finding Common Ground Within the Partnership**, the reader will be able to:

- Describe effective strategies for promoting and maintaining trust, communication, connectedness, respect, and meaningful work.
- Identify effective processes for resolving conflict and finding common ground within the research partnership.

Introduction

After the initial preparatory and relationship-building work has been accomplished, the research team moves into the next phase of project work, which consists of dealing with day-to-day challenges to the work and partnership. A great deal of time and effort was spent by researchers on gaining entry into the community and building relationships of mutual trust and respect. With this strong foundation in place, ongoing work now centers on maintaining and strengthening the partnership.

Researchers must establish a safe environment for community partners to voice their concerns and opinions. They must concentrate their efforts on constantly monitoring the relationship to ensure that imbalances of power and influence do not develop, much less permeate the research environment. At this stage in the process, partners must pay close attention to methods used to handle conflict and disagreement within the group, and to maintaining the strong, healthy relationship that they have worked so hard to build.

How Do Researchers Determine the Values and Needs of the Community?

Understanding and respecting a community's values and needs are paramount in conducting a successful CBPR study. However, CBPR researchers recognize early on that it is *only* by developing a meaningful, honest relationship that they can truly understand the community's values and needs. Developing such a relationship usually takes a great deal of time and effort and may not work within the limitations of agency funding and other project resources. Be sure to understand the potential CBPR timeline, and that early relationship-building with a community may need to be started well in advance of applying for research funding.

As relationship-building progresses, researchers will be made keenly aware of the state of mental healthcare resources within the community. Those who are familiar with the realities of community-based organizations (CBOs) and other nonprofit healthcare settings understand how such groups must consistently find ways to do more to benefit the local community, often with inadequate or dwindling resources. Peoplepower and funding are often in such short supply that the only option available is simply to do less. Research can benefit a community by providing a way for it to work more effectively using fewer resources. Again, this process requires that a relationship exists in which researchers truly understand the existing situations and resulting community needs.

A CBPR project creates new information that has the potential to help make the work of community-based mental health providers more effective. Community-based research can produce valuable information that is tailored to the community studied and addresses its unique concerns. Further, the CBPR study, within the study protocol, often provides valuable treatment services to community members that would not otherwise be available.

Partnering with Community-Based Agencies

Even though a community may enthusiastically embrace the possibility of entering into a CBPR project, enthusiasm alone does not ensure a smooth process. Time is often a major concern. For example, community mental health agencies typically cannot afford to allow their employees time away from their duties for outside research work. One strategy to lessen this barrier is to find ways to weave research project activities into the tasks of CBO staff and volunteers. For example, volunteers calling on patients in the community might incorporate a satisfaction or needs survey into these visits, which can be designed to provide valuable information to both the local agency and the CBPR team. Researchers can volunteer to work side by side with agency staff, contributing their expertise to agency efforts while gaining firsthand knowledge that contributes to their understanding of the needs of the community. These partnerships can provide critical insight into the community that increases understanding of local mental health concerns, and of the contextual factors that affects all aspects of the study.

Paying Attention to Local Media

In addition to working closely with CBOs, researchers can gain another layer of understanding by reading local newspapers, newsletters, or other periodicals. These publications may contain human interest articles and features about local groups, organizations, projects, and "real people" that are important to the community. They may provide important contact information for follow-up, insights into community culture, and an "invitation" into the stories of community members whom the research team might otherwise never know. Not only is this strategy helpful early in project planning, but it may also provide a method for maintaining and strengthening the research relationship. Any method researchers can find to demonstrate genuine interest and caring about community life will serve to strengthen the bond between partners.

Engaging in Brainstorming Sessions

Another approach to gaining information about needs and values is to engage in brainstorming sessions with community members. Researchers and members gather in groups that are a manageable size so all participants have the opportunity to contribute. In the brainstorming sessions, a member of the research team should be responsible for note-taking on all topics and issues addressed. The note-taker should not edit information gathered during the session, but simply record all comments. Once information is organized and lists are complete, researchers may begin to see overlap or frequently mentioned issues that can be addressed in the research work. Activities such as this help researchers stay in contact with the larger community, rather than relying too heavily on a few select community representatives and missing the perspectives and opinions of the community-at-large. Keep in mind that if the research team decides to audiorecord or videotape the discussion, all those attending the meeting must provide consent.

Establishing a Community Resource Inventory

An outside research team can also consider conducting a community resource inventory to help identify needs. A resource inventory helps to determine the extent to which currently existing mental health resources are meeting community mental health needs. In some CBPR projects, the research team brings together a core group of community representatives with knowledge about the current state of local mental health care. This group collaborates with the research team to create a shared understanding of the community's mental health needs, and to determine how well and to what extent existing resources are meeting those needs. Examining local mental health treatment resources provides an additional layer of information for the research partners to understand existing community needs, and to use when evaluating or adjusting project progress, focus, and goals.

Over the course of the CBPR project, it is crucial that researchers keep their work focused primarily on community benefit. The ultimate goal of CBPR is always to provide benefit to the community. Research alone is not sufficient to achieve this goal. It is the integration of scientific research and community values, culture, and needs that makes CBPR a unique and useful research strategy.

Researcher Reflection

What are the advantages for community members who participate in a study?

One study of family resiliency looked at how we were doing over a course of about 5 years. That was through the Beach Center. And it was really interesting for me thinking early on how we've got it all together and things aren't that bad, when our littlest guy, who has multiple disabilities, was getting early intervention services. Life was pretty good; we thought it was always going to be like that. But as he got older and the system of service changed, it got harder to access the same level of care. And the people, the player changed so much more rapidly, and in the school district and in private therapy that we did start to see that it was getting harder for us to keep all the threads together. And so being asked those questions again over a period of years really helped me see as a family that our life had gotten a lot more complex. As our child's needs were more clearly known as he got older and it became pretty obvious he was going to have severe impairments.

Excerpted from a video interview with Cheryl Scott, Parent Navigator Training Coordinator, Anchorage, Alaska

Scientists must have genuine respect for their community partners - they must trust that their partners will let them know when they're wrong, and won't let the study move in the wrong direction.

How Are Implicit Concerns Expressed?

Building and maintaining the relationships necessary for CBPR require a blend of science, professionalism, and humanism. Researchers possessing scientific knowledge and a strong sense of logic have the tools they need to conduct a traditional research with acceptable levels of validity and reliability, but compassion, patience, empathy, openness, and understanding are additional tools needed to conduct successful CBPR. Researchers and community partners must be able to successfully develop a research environment in which all partners feel valued and respected, and are free to voice their thoughts, opinions, and concerns.

The work of the CBPR partners must continuously be monitored for imbalances in power and influence. Although power differentials may exist outside of the partnership, researchers must ensure that those imbalances do not enter into the working relationship. When the team is involved in CBPR project work, equality among all partners must be respected and maintained.

Hierarchy

Communities are seldom a neat, cohesive single unit. Rather, they have internal groups of power and influence along with their subgroups. Researchers must be aware of the internal dynamics and the history of the community and its subgroups. There needs to be an awareness of the hierarchies currently in place, and the subgroups that in the past have not had their voices heard. Researchers must not allow the influence of these issues to impact the study, while remaining mindful of current and historical imbalances of power and influence. By understanding community power structures, both past and present, researchers can more successfully achieve true representativeness of the study sample, and accurate interpretation of study data and results.

Dialogue

It is important that community dialogue includes all levels of diversity and representation. Daniel Yankelovich (1999) defines dialogue as a verbal interaction (conversation) for the purpose of increasing understanding between those engaged in the interaction. Yankelovich believes that the process of dialogue must include the following elements:

- Equal participation
- Voluntary, noncoercive exchanges

- Empathic listening
- Surfacing of assumptions

According to Yankelovich, if all four elements are not present in the interaction, it should not be considered a dialogue. When true dialogue within the community is taking place, individuals who have felt marginalized in the past will be able to name and define their own experiences and needs. All aspects of community diversity must have a voice in the process in order for the work to speak to the true scope of community needs.

Equitable Partnership

Efforts to maintain equity among community partners and members must be ongoing. Researchers must actively seek out broad scope community representation by finding ways to hear all its voices—from the most to the least powerful. Although the research team may be doing all it can to promote equality among the individuals involved in the study, community members also exist alongside each other outside of project work. It may be difficult for them to "switch gears" in their relationships. Since some community members may not feel free to contribute thoughts or opinions in an open forum, it is important for researchers to offer a number of "safe" communication options, such as e-mail, suggestion boxes, and opportunities for one-on-one discussions, which are reviewed in Chapter 5. These alternatives may help increase participation by community members who want to be heard but do not feel free to speak out publicly. Providing other means of communication will help ensure that the study includes a broad scope of community perspectives, input, and participation including those who have had little or no influence in the past.

How Do Partners Find Common Ground on Differing Goals and Preferences?

One of the best ways to ensure that research partners share common ground from the beginning is to develop mutually created goals, guidelines, and processes during the initial phases of the project.

These parameters must reflect the basic principles of CBPR. Carrying out project work within these guidelines must take place in an atmosphere that fosters the following ways of being healthy:

- Openness
- Patience
- Caring
- Attentive, active listening
- Respect
- Trust
- Agreement to disagree
- Equality
- Nonjudgment of others' perspectives and opinions
- Seeing value in diverse perspectives
- Compromise
- Support of all team members' contributions
- Sensitivity to diversity
- Acceptance

Of particular importance are operating guidelines that promote understanding and sensitivity to diversity within the group and the larger community (e.g., gender, social standing, education, age, and race). As procedures and guidelines are created and adjusted throughout the process, it is necessary to keep in mind that they cannot be *imposed* upon the partners, but rather they must be *co-created* and mutually agreed upon by the very group they are meant to organize.

At every stage of the project work, open dialogue is essential. It serves as a tool to reach mutual understanding—leading to unity of purpose within a group. It also provides a decision-making aid for people coming together with diverse experiences, views, and values.

What Are the Processes for Dealing with Conflicts and Disagreements on an Ongoing Basis?

When a diverse group of individuals joins together to work as a cohesive group and develop a single, shared vision, disagreement is likely to emerge. Disagreement about decisions related to project work among the partners must not be viewed as a problem or a sign of ineffectiveness, but rather as an opportunity for sharing from all partners. Indeed, such disagreement may be a sign that all partners feel sufficiently involved and safe to voice their own opinions with assertiveness and without fear of reprisal. Disagreements can also be viewed as a way for researchers to demonstrate their commitment to *really listening* to the ideas and concerns of the community. It is in taking a truly respectful, participatory approach to disagreement that all partners recognize they are operating in a safe environment in which every voice is heard and valued.

Researchers must always assume that there is a legitimate reason for conflict; it is never productive to seek out a troublemaker or attempt to lay blame. If serious conflict occurs, the research team must make the time to resolve it before moving ahead with the next project task. When handled properly, conflict can provide the research team with an opportunity for constructive growth and change, and it can demonstrate conflict resolution and effective compromise for the greater community.

The following are a few simple approaches for lessening or resolving conflict (Center for Collaborative Planning 2002). These are not the only means to resolve conflict but are useful first steps.

Approaches to Conflict

- *Facilitated group discussions.* Group discussions on the diversity of personality, perspective, assumptions, race, ethnicity, culture, language, and training that exists among members can help ease conflict. Group communication needs to be implicitly and explicitly sensitive to the cultural differences in individual approaches to communicating, disclosing, decision-making, and conflict resolution.
- *Immediacy of conflict resolution.* Differences of style, opinion, approach, or process within the group need to be discussed and resolved as they arise. Any conflicts ignored by the group are bound to resurface later with increased intensity.
- *Openness and nonjudgment.* The research team must create an atmosphere within the group wherein all members are comfortable with their right to bring up issues and have them resolved to everyone's satisfaction.
- *Roots of the problem.* Researchers need to identify the probable causes of conflicts that emerge, such as lack of information, power struggles or competition for control, personality conflict, and loss of direction. Only if the root of the problem is correctly identified will the team be able to find the right solution.

Too much time is wasted in conflict resolution when the group works on a symptom rather than the underlying cause.

- *Identification of mutually acceptable solutions.* The research team does well to negotiate solutions by hearing all sides of an issue and focusing on common ground that may emerge in these discussions. If a conflict is long-standing and entrenched, it may be wise for the research team to consider hiring a third party or mediator to assist with facilitating conflict resolution so the researchers do not become identified with it.
- *Explicit contract.* A successful negotiation is best capped off with an explicit agreement about what was decided. Once the group has developed a contract (whether written or verbal), it also needs a commensurate process to monitor contract adherence by all partners.

As the research team moves through the project work, group cohesiveness increases and work efficiencies begin to develop. Efficiency must not translate into complacency or indifference. Instead, research team members, as they monitor group processes, need to keep in mind the complexity of the group's functioning for the entire project duration. They must remain aware at all times that groups function in multiple ways including, but not limited to, the following possibilities.

- *Social function.* During the relationship-building phase, researchers and community partners often form personal as well as working relationships which help create an environment of trust and sharing. Social relationships among partners can be strengthened by engaging in social or team-building activities outside of project work.
- *Task-completion function.* Research partners are charged with the task of working together to conduct scientific research that will benefit the community. At times it may be helpful to create small, task-oriented subgroups to complete specific tasks that arise during project work.
- *Information-sharing function.* Research team members meet to inform, to be informed, and to clarify goals, provide input on the process, and consider other perspectives in making adjustments to the process. Ongoing information-sharing among partners is important in keeping the project on track.
- *Learning function.* The group meets to improve skills or increase knowledge among partners through information-sharing.

What If the Partnership Fails?

CBPR researchers may be under the assumption that every research partnership will succeed. However, there may be circumstances under which it is appropriate to allow a partnership to end. Although many research relationships between communities and professional or academic institutions develop into long-term affiliations, some come to a natural end when the project is completed, or when another purpose of the partnership has been fulfilled. Others may not end on good terms, ceasing abruptly with one or more of the partners dissatisfied. Knowing how to determine when a partnership should end can be difficult and stressful for all involved partners. Having the skills to know how to negotiate an end to the partnership needs to be part of the CBPR researcher's toolbox.

To be able to negotiate endings, researchers need to be aware of the reasons why partnerships terminate, some of which are listed below (Israel et al. 1998). There may be other reasons for a partnership to end. Keep in mind that each CBPR partnership is unique. This book provides guidelines, but each study must be managed according to its unique features and qualities.

Common Reasons CBPR Partnerships End

- Upon completion of targeted goals; when the study is finished
- Cases of dishonesty, misuse, or abuse within the partnership
- When there are inadequate resources to support the partnership (in some cases, this may be a temporary termination, with agreement to come together again if a funding source or key personnel is identified)
- When there has been a gross violation of the partnership's principles

When these or other circumstances occur and any of the partners consider ending the relationship, a number of questions should be discussed and answered (Israel et al. 1998).

- How will partners know whether the partnership should end versus when it just needs to be fixed?

- What are the benefits and drawbacks to ending the relationship from the perspectives of all partners?
- When is it okay to end a relationship?
- Are there any available resources within the community or the research team to address the problems or strengthen weaknesses in the partnership?
- What are the partners willing to sacrifice to maintain the relationship?
- What are the partners *not* willing to sacrifice to maintain the relationship?

What Ethical Safeguards Does the Community Need or Want?

Community partners contribute valuable information and insights to the participatory research process. This being said, there is an assumption on the part of the community that researchers will use their professional expertise and knowledge to conduct their work with the highest degree of professionalism with regard to scientific rigor and ethical treatment of study participants. To ensure that the community's trust in the research team is protected and expectations are met, a number of issues must be considered.

As discussed in Chapter 3, there are systems in place to protect *individual* participants from harm when involved in research studies in general, and in clinical trials in particular. However, no formal guidelines exist to protect *groups* involved in research studies conducted in community settings. Some investigators may believe that the safeguards for research with individuals can simply be transferred to groups in community settings, but this is not as easy as it seems, and it is not an adequate, responsible solution.

As new models for and approaches to CBPR emerge, ethical guidelines and participant safeguards must be developed to protect both individuals and groups within the greater community. CBPR researchers are often challenged with finding common ground with partners as they consider community perspectives and needs while incorporating established human protections guidelines in research. This topic raises a number of points that need to be addressed by the research team, some of which are discussed below.

IRB Review

In order to address the safeguards that honor the needs of the community, each study protocol should undergo regular reviews by both an institutional review board (IRB) and a community review board. Community reviews are often conducted by the Community Advisory Board (CAB) that may be in place, or was formed specifically for the study. In other cases, research teams develop an entirely new board that has as its purpose the oversight of research work, with particular focus on how each step of the study adheres to the ethics and human protection guidelines agreed upon early in the process by the research partners, the IRB, and possibly the CAB. Often, boards specifically created to oversee the work of a study are referred to as Data Safety and Monitoring Boards (DSMB).

This dual process keeps the issue of human protection at the forefront of both the institutional requirements of the research team and community protections. It also helps to maintain a community voice in the process when the research team is using an IRB that does not have members with CBPR training or adequate knowledge of the principles of CBPR. The IRB and the community review board should explore ways to collaborate on the review process, such as having representatives or liaisons between boards to communicate and coordinate review activities.

Research Agreement

To ensure that community partners and the community-at-large are protected from harm resulting from participation in the study, the research partnership must have a written research agreement in place. This agreement should be developed, approved, and signed by all involved parties. Developed collaboratively, before project planning begins, the research agreement must be considered a living document, changed or adjusted in response to new knowledge gained during the research process. This will accommodate changes in personnel or other resources, changes in the political climate within the community, and new insights shared by partners and the greater community over the life of the project. The research agreement contributes to the validity of the work and minimizes harm and maximizes benefits to the community.

It also creates a protection plan for partners if the relationship should fail. Research agreements must address, in detail, every aspect of the partnership and the project work, from planning to dissemination or application of results. Some important questions that can guide creation of the research agreement are:

- *Protection of the individual and the community.* Does the document protect the anonymity and/or confidentiality of research volunteers? Does it protect the confidentiality of the community? Are individuals protected from irresponsibility or wrongdoing within the partnership? Are the project description, goals, timelines, and objectives written in collaboration, or at least in agreement with community partners? Specifically, how will decision-making and conflict resolution be handled? In detail, how are responsibilities shared or divided? Who will serve as decision-maker if the group is divided?
- *Interfacing the community and the IRB.* What process is in place for the community review board to evaluate and approve proposed research and changes to the protocol in tandem with the IRB? How will final decisions regarding safeguards and protections be handled when there is conflict or disagreement between the groups? Does the IRB contain members with CBPR knowledge or training, or will a community representative be selected to join the board?
- *Jurisdiction and ownership.* To what extent does each group have jurisdiction over data, data interpretation, and dissemination of results? Who will ultimately own the data and will they be made available in any form to other researchers? If so, how will confidentiality be protected? How will results be translated into community benefit? Who will be responsible for implementation of community change?

When working in communities, it is important to be mindful of issues such as stigmatization of individuals with mental health issues, self-stigmatization, and the amount of community disruption caused by the project work. Project guidelines regarding safeguards for individuals and the community must reflect the research with respect to local culture, values, and needs, and should reflect collaboration of knowledge and perspectives between researchers and community partners. When handled professionally and in keeping with the principles of CBPR, safeguard guidelines can strengthen the relationship as trust continues to be built between researchers and the community.

Researcher Reflection

How is information about a study communicated to community members?

Well typically we would first hear about a study through a service provider, or through another family, or in the early days through hard copy newsletters. Then if it seemed like something of interest, we'd contact whoever it was and if we fit the demographic they were looking for then they would sign us up. There had even been a couple of times where things were done in Canada and they were having such a hard time getting people that fit the population they wanted to use that I would get a call back a couple months later saying, we've decided to expand our focus and we are now looking at the northern shield including Alaska, not just Canada, in order to try to get enough people to participate. So, once we would actually be involved a packet would come in the mail or it would be faxed to me that would have release forms and it would explain what the purpose of the research study was for and how our confidentiality would be protected and I always really appreciated that I could share that information and I could tell them what I was comfortable sharing publicly and what I didn't want [to] be counted as part of the aggregate. So I really liked those studies where they did all that ahead of time. That was the first thing I heard about and also to know why...What was going to be the long term benefit for our family participating in this? Because it usually took a fair amount of time filling out paperwork, or doing phone interviews, or occasionally face-to-face conversations, so it was nice to know about how much time was going to be asked of us.

Excerpted from a video interview with Cheryl Scott, Parent Navigator Training Coordinator, Anchorage, Alaska

What Are the Jurisdiction Issues?

The CBPR principle of creating an equal partnership between researchers and the community may initially be met with skepticism as early community engagement takes place. In traditional research, which many communities have already experienced, often evident power differentials and an inequitable distribution of power and control occur between researchers and the community. Past power and influence differentials may have centered on issues such as race, ethnicity, education level, class, and gender. In past experiences with traditional research, communities may have perceived an absence of control in the process.

Researchers hoping to work with communities face the important task of convincing potential partners that they will share authority in all decision-making, from defining the research question, to conducting the study, to dealing with the results. Community partners need to be convinced that they own the process and the outcomes of the study, and that the most important goal of the work is to produce important information that will benefit the community and improve the lives of its members.

Funding is a practical reality of any research endeavor. In an attempt to satisfy requirements of the project's funding sources, some imbalances may be created in regard to who holds the authority and control over the work. Researchers should constantly check their motivation, to ensure that they are not becoming more funding-driven than project-driven. Being funding-driven refers to having an overall goal of obtaining financial support even if it means that original or current project work must be adjusted or changed to fit the funding agency requirements. Such a strategy can harm a CBPR study in the long run. Although being funding-driven results in financial support for ongoing project work, it can also distract from the partnership and take time and energy away from previously identified goals and priorities that were named with community input. If funding becomes the project's main driving force, many CBPR principles will be lost and the community may turn its back on the research.

Example:

Although every effort was made to develop equity in the partnership, community members noted a definite power differential around issues of money. Since the university applied for and received project funding, the scientific team served as fiscal agent with very little money coming directly to the community.

In order to mobilize the community for project work and beyond, community needs should be written into grant budgets, or community partners employed in the grant-writing process.

In contrast, project-driven research teams seek out funding that fits with previously determined research aims and goals. For the authority and control of a project to remain in the hands of community partners, researchers must design a long-term funding plan in which the community-stated project focus remains the top priority. In order to address any funding-related skepticism about equity among partners, there are increasing numbers of funding initiatives that not only allow, but require that project funds are directly paid to community partners. As funding agencies become more familiar with participatory research, new funding strategies are being created. Researchers can seek out 1-year planning grants designed to fund the planning/relationship-building stages of a proposed study. Other types of grants are designed to direct money straight to the community. Research teams can also establish procedures for subcontracting with CBOs for their services. Whatever terms of funding have been arranged, both community partners and researchers must understand, early on, the details of their accounting responsibilities for project funds.

Researcher Reflection

How do you address multiple agenda issues?

Typically you have funding restraints in terms of when the report or the project is to be completed; and so as a researcher, you're under pressure to get things done in a particular time frame. I don't think that sense of urgency is always the same for the community partners. It also becomes real difficult as you're engaging community partners when they've got to provide input or respond to something. Oftentimes it takes a long time to get them to do their piece and yet you can't move forward without their piece. There's times when we basically had to just say we are not going to get it and move forward. But that is absolutely a critical one, I don't have any good answers for that other than to again remind people that there are timelines and where the pressure points are.

Excerpted from a video interview with Karen Ward, Ph.D., Professor and Director, Center for Human Development, University of Alaska Anchorage

Case Study 4.1

The academic researchers, having little experience or relationship with the rural community partners, were finding that trust-building was an arduous process. The team not only spent a considerable amount of time discussing, authoring, and adopting a specific, detailed set of CBPR principles and ground rules, but also developed additional rules and operating norms to help the group adhere to these principles. One of their strategies was to use group consensus in all decision-making. The group decided that they would apply a 75 percent rule to guide their work, rather than simply using majority rule. They decided that using consensus would lead to group discussions and debates of divisive topics. When the group discussed or debated an issue, they found that they shared more perspectives, people brought support for their point of view, and often quieter, less vocal partners contributed their thoughts and ideas. As the project work progressed, the partners reflected on the process. They collectively felt that once consensus was reached on an issue, all partners were more informed on the topic and overall more satisfied with the group decision. While community partners identify this process as contributing to equity and shared influence, the drawback is that it often takes a considerable amount of time.

Important Issues to Address

- What are the community's expectations when the partners are divided on an issue?
- How do you maintain pace with project timelines (academic, funding, community) while respecting all perspectives on an issue where the community or the research team is divided?
- How will partners respond when consensus or common ground cannot be reached on an issue?
- How can the research team ensure that scientific rigor is preserved in decision-making without being perceived as authoritative?

Case Study 4.2

During the initial phases of the project, researchers worked closely with the director of a local community-based organization (CBO). The director had been an active part of the project from the start, and was instrumental in helping researchers build trust in the community. She also aided in recruiting participants into the study by identifying community leaders, facilitating town meetings, and contributing meeting space, her time, and staff to various study-related activities. Early in the second year of project, the relationship between the director and the CBO board became strained over their differing perspectives regarding how to expand the organization's community services. The director was interested in extending the breadth of services to people living in more remote, outlying areas. The board was interested in increasing the depth of services to community residents residing in close proximity to the center. The conflict affected the research agenda indirectly because it placed increased demands on the director's time, reducing her availability for research activities. Also, the conflict led to each side taking an all-or-nothing attitude in their positions on the issue. Eventually, the sides became gridlocked and the director was forced to relinquish her position with the organization. Despite the track record of the research team and its work with the community, the project was closely associated with the former director and did not receive support from the board. Consequently, the project was put on hold and the researchers were compelled to seek other CBO support.

Important Issues to Address

- How diverse is the scope of community representation in the partnership?
- How will the partnership survive if community or other obligations interfere with the commitments of its membership?
- How are tasks and responsibilities distributed among research partners?
- Have all partners' strengths and talents been recognized? Where is the overlap (if any)?
- How will tasks and responsibilities be handled if a partner leaves the partnership?

Case Study 4.3

The director of a community health clinic contacted university researchers with the request to develop a community-based participatory research (CBPR) project in response to a research grant solicitation. Over the next few months, the director and staff worked closely with the researchers to develop a mutually acceptable plan. Special efforts were made to ensure a high level of local involvement, including the development of a position for a full-time, on-site project coordinator. The grant was submitted, funded, and the project was initiated. Throughout the first year, all activities were completed to the satisfaction of all participants. At the start of year 2, the directorship of the clinic changed. The new director began to implement plans for a greatly expanded sphere of activities, including plans for creating a national research center in the community. New staff positions were created and long-standing staff members were reassigned or left the agency. The new director announced that protocols for existing research activities and management of all grant-supported staff needed to change in order to allow the new research center to assume full control of the scope of work and ownership of all products generated by the CBPR. The director expected that the funding agency would remove the grant from the university and award it to the community research center. Rather than a collaborative effort, decisions would be made by the research center management team.

Important Issues to Address

- What are the mechanisms and rules for funding?
- What are the expectations for partners?
- Could a comprehensive research agreement at the start of the partnership have prevented these problems?
- Are there ethical concerns that could influence the integrity of the CBPR?

Case Study 4.4

A group of researchers entered a community to help with resource development centered on recent increases in domestic violence, perhaps secondary to an economic downturn after closure of a major local industry. They engaged in formative work, networking with various stakeholder groups to clarify the issues, identify desired outcomes, and develop acceptable interventions and prevention activities. In meetings with various stakeholder groups (city officials, former employers, unemployed men, affected families, and social service and healthcare providers), the researchers became keenly aware of many divergent ways of thinking about the issues among these various groups and unearthed long-standing resentments and lingering anger that had developed many years before. Most importantly, they identified that the unemployed men and the former employer had strongly divergent views of the need for the shutdown of the company and that the conflict between these groups had developed several year prior. The researchers also discovered that the employer had strong ties into the home lives of its employees pre-closure in that it often awarded bonuses based on factors external to the work and more related to family circumstances of the men. One value that was clearly expressed by the employer through financial incentives was large families with stay-at-home mothers. This value had seeped into local family life and had greatly affected spousal relationships. Post-closure family dynamics shifted rapidly and unexpectedly and much anger developed across different stakeholder groups. The anger across stakeholder groups emerged loudly in every stakeholder meeting with the researchers and had derailed the research process regularly and with many hard feelings on both the community and researcher side. At this point, the researchers were considering pulling out of the community due to the belief that emotions were running too high and people were too antagonized for the research team to enter the community effectively.

Important Issues to Address

- How can researchers deal with meetings that generate a lot of strong affect across stakeholder groups and directed at the research team?

- How can researchers work to identify false dichotomies across groups?
- What are some effective ways to help groups develop openness toward compromise?
- Do researchers have a role or responsibility in mediating conflict between diverse stakeholder groups?
- How can stakeholder groups with diverse opinions and strong affects be brought to the same table?
- What are the ethical implications of researchers opening up a conversation in a community and then abandoning the community because emotions run high?

Chapter 5
Sustaining the Partnership

Upon completion of **Chapter 5: Sustaining the Partnership**, the reader will be able to:

- Apply strategies to build, sustain, and strengthen the community partnership.
- Identify and synthesize strategies to monitor and maintain equality of power and influence within the partnership.

Introduction

As the work of a CBPR project ensues, the partnership may, at times, lose sight of the overarching purpose of the project—creating or contributing to lasting, positive community change. This goal can only be achieved when outside researchers partner as *equals* with the community working toward a shared vision. Although it seems as though it should be relatively easy to sustain equality within the partnership, day-to-day issues often arise that become roadblocks to the process.

In addition to laying the proper foundation for the research, ongoing attention must be paid to the researchers' relationship with the community and its members, and to the processes involved in carrying out the study. Balance of power, equality of voice, and appropriate community representation must be monitored every step of the way. Research team members must continue to value community input and opinion as the primary influence on changes or adjustments to the process. In addition,

L.W. Roberts, *Community-Based Participatory Research for Improved Mental Healthcare*, DOI 10.1007/978-1-4614-5517-2_5, © Springer Science+Business Media New York 2013 researchers must be ever mindful of the ultimate goal of increasing community capacity to produce and maintain real and lasting change when the study is complete. For the project to be truly successful, project work should be created and produced collaboratively with the very people who are *most likely* to benefit from the results.

Chapter 5 focuses on strategies researchers can use to sustain the partnership that they have formed with the community, and to monitor how closely the study process adheres to the principles of participatory research.

Researcher Reflection

Why should CBPR be viewed as a long-term process?

Community based research is a long process, so when we came to a system we weren't saying, well, this is one little project that we want to do and if we can't do it the way we want to do it, then there's just no point. We had to look at…thinking we want to develop a relationship with you as a system so that we start here. But ten years from now we're still going to be working together and we're still going to be doing things that are going to be benefiting people inside prison and out. So, I have to take the long-term view on this and look at what's possible to do now and realize that, 4 or 5 years down the road, that is, I've been a good collaborator with you and I've been worthy of being trusted, I think that's a real critical term. If you can trust me as a scientist to come in and do my best work, within the limits and boundaries that you set, then over time, those limits and boundaries change. And that's part of thinking long term.

Excerpted from a video interview with Gloria Eldridge, Ph.D., Associate Professor of Psychology, University of Alaska Anchorage

---

How Are Day-to-Day Issues Addressed?

The everyday issues that are likely to arise during the study should not present a great deal of difficulty if, during the initial phase, researchers and community partners collaboratively determined a well-thought out and detailed research agreement, or at the very least developed a project plan. Although creating the initial plan or agreement is certain to require some time and adjustment, if well-thought out, it will provide a guide for decision-making throughout the study, and a reference for solving day-to-day issues and questions that are inherent in the participatory process.

Adjustments to the Process

As noted earlier in this book, many decisions made in the initial planning phase may need to be adjusted due to the cyclic, reflective nature of CBPR. As new knowledge is gained through information-sharing between partners, the process may require modification. Also, new ways of doing things may evolve based on group discussions and reflections as the process unfolds. Traditional researchers are typically not used to a model in which they are asked to react to data before a study is complete. More often than not, traditional research relies on the full body of data being collected before reviewing findings and interpreting data.

CBPR is, therefore, best viewed as a study in which the research partners look at data every step of the way. Ongoing review and analysis often provide the stimulus for adjustments to the research process. This process is similar to that in a clinical drug trial with an active data safety monitoring board that can react to research findings early on—and can either stop the study altogether or ask that a particularly useful drug be made available to the control group. In CBPR, the research partners function somewhat as a data safety monitoring board by reviewing the process from a community perspective, and scrutinizing and interpreting data as they are collected, with authority to recommend adjustments based on the new information. It is important that as such adjustments occur, all partners are in agreement about how and when to implement them. It is critical to maintain a balance in decision-making between scientific rigor and community benefit.

Communication with Diverse Audiences

Throughout a CBPR study, researchers hold meetings and discussions to keep community members updated about what is happening in the research process, the status of current activities, and the direction for future work. These meetings also provide opportunities for people to voice their opinions. To ensure that communication efforts are respectful and understandable by all, researchers may need to alter their presentation style to suit different groups. For example, if the community-at-large is addressed, a presentation may need to be markedly different than one designed for members or leaders of community-based organizations (CBOs), who may not reflect the overall community, particularly in terms of educational level, income, community status, and/or perspective.

Input into many aspects of the research process and decisions about issues should ideally come from a broad range of community representatives, not just a select group. Although it is not practical to involve each member of the community in every project-related decision, large group updates and Q&A sessions are important in maintaining trust and involvement with the community. To this end, the research team must find ways to reach all levels of the community and provide opportunities for interested parties to contribute. As mentioned in Chapter 4, offering a range of communication options helps to promote increased participation in the research process. Some examples of communication options follow.

Open meetings with facilitated group discussions provide a communication platform for a large number of people. However, community members who have conflicts with the day and time of a scheduled meeting or who are not comfortable making public comments may need an alternate type of forum.

Creative solutions help to assure that all community members are invited to participate in the process and that their voices will be heard, such as:

- A choice of small group discussion times
- A block of time during which community members can drop by to meet with the research team
- Scheduled one-on-one meetings with researchers
- Town hall discussions, ideal for giving less-involved community members a voice in the process
- Open-ended surveys
- Confidential e-mail communication with researchers
- Community blogs
- Suggestion boxes

Researchers may achieve the best results when they ask community partners to provide suggestions for effective ways to communicate with the community-at-large. Regardless of the strategies chosen, the goal is to assure that gathering input results in an accurate and wide representation of community opinions.

The communication methods used by the research team to handle day-to-day issues help to ensure the success of the participatory effort. By experiencing the effects of having an important and valued voice in decisions made by the research team, community partners learn to trust the process and feel empowered to create real and lasting community change.

> Because we were committed to a process that was *participatory*, and we related leadership to power, we were unwilling to assert much leadership with community partners. After reflecting on the process, we found that we had inadvertently marginalized ourselves.

How Is Equality of All Partners Maintained Throughout the Process?

Research teams entering a community must remain mindful that they are conducting research *with* people, not *on* people. When a true participatory approach is used, the individuals included in the study are also involved in many aspects of the research project. When a community shares control of the process with the research team and maintains an equally powerful voice, a few power issues come into play. It is important to remember that the more collective and participatory the process is at each step, the more likely the outcome will reflect the uniqueness of the community and will have meaning to the individuals who are most affected by results.

Importance of Interpersonal Skills

In addition to the need for researchers to be knowledgeable about and skilled in research techniques, they must also be personable and able to engage community partners. With a solid base of interpersonal skills, goodwill, empathy, understanding, and the capacity to relate to others in a meaningful way (without arrogance or superiority), researchers will be able to connect on a personal level with community members.

Throughout the CBPR process, research team members need to maintain their proper place in the community, or they will risk destroying the trust and rapport built during the initial phases of the study. One of the biggest mistakes researchers can make is to be engaging and inviting early on as the community is being wooed, and then turn away as the project work begins. This scenario paves a rapid path to communities feeling used and manipulated and is completely contrary to CBPR principles. Indeed, many historical cases of failed community-based research developed exactly in this manner—researchers were invited into a community after initially presenting a collaborative or cooperative stance, only to ignore or shut the community out during project work or after the data were collected and interpreted.

Understanding Roles

Engaging a community in every step of the process is sometimes interpreted by traditional researchers as a situation in which they must leave behind their professional standards, experience, and knowledge, and rely on the community to steer the entire process. This is not what CBPR is about. CBPR involves each member of the partnership, whether researcher or community member, sharing her or his own unique gifts while accepting the gifts of others through a reciprocal learning process.

It may be as difficult for scientific researchers to let go of their roles as research "experts" as it is for the community partners to let go of their roles of patient, client, and so on. For each member of the research partnership, letting go of old conceptions of who they are may require private and public self-reflection about sources of power in their own lives and how personal and social history might influence the work of the partnership. The areas in which research partners may need to self-reflect include the following:

- Scientific members remind themselves to value nonscientific voices that speak from great experience and community knowledge.
- Community members remind themselves to value expert research and methodological voices that speak from academic learning.
- Partners recognize and address any negative or mistrustful feelings they have toward others in the partnership.
- Old hierarchical patterns of both the researchers and community members are acknowledged, and new roles and structure are created as research partners learn to examine their interactions.

The effectiveness of the partnership will increase if all members share responsibility for identifying and monitoring patterns of interpersonal conduct in a respectful, collaborative manner that reflects equality and caring. This process clearly supports the critical CBPR principle of equity among the research partners.

Ensuring equal voice is the responsibility of the scientific members of the research team, at least initially. There are several helpful strategies researchers can use to ensure that the process remains true to CBPR principles.

Strategies for Ensuring Equality

- *Self-monitoring of value systems*. Every researcher brings to the process his or her personal assumptions and biases based on individual value systems. Thus, procedures should be developed and put in place for each researcher to self-monitor to ensure that personal issues are not influencing the work of the team, and that he or she is not imposing personal values and assumptions onto the community. Also, researchers may feel a constant struggle between thinking that they know what is best for a community and being overly cautious to not contribute their perspective out of fear of having too much influence. In such cases, a frank and open discussion among the research partners is usually the best course of action.
- *Monitoring the community relationship*. The relationship between researchers and community members should be constantly monitored and nurtured by the research team to

ensure that community partners are not taken for granted. This requires ongoing reflection on the health of the partnership. Trust and respect are dynamic and can waiver if not given steady and sustained attention. Since CBPR involves human beings interacting with each other as equal partners, it depends on a delicate balance of give and take. It is important to monitor this relationship for indications of even the slightest imbalance, particularly if the shift begins to swing power to the research team. If the relationship becomes seriously imbalanced, parties on both sides will feel it and respond on some level even if that reaction is not apparent to others. Keep in mind, however, imbalance is not always negative. If it does occur, the researchers should acknowledge the imbalance and focus on minimizing its impact and duration. For example, a temporary imbalance may occur in a decision-making situation that finds scientific and community partners in disagreement. When such a case occurs, researchers may want to defer to the perspective of community partners to ensure ongoing positive feelings and commitment to the study. After periods of imbalance or disagreement, and also during times of agreement and cooperation, the research team should find opportunities to comment on how much they have learned during the process and how greatly the science and process of the study are strengthened by using a co-learning approach.

• *Evaluating the process.* Another way to monitor the equity status within the partnership is to regularly gather input and comments from everyone involved on how they feel the study is going. Such ongoing evaluations can take the form of discussions, interviews, open meetings, surveys, and open-ended questionnaires. Encouraging widespread community participation in study evaluations increases the effectiveness of the partnership, communicates to community members that their voices are being heard and are valued, and keeps the process in line with the cyclic and iterative nature of CBPR.

The path to a successful CBPR study is clear—the more participation and collaboration, the better. If researchers engage and involve the community at every step of the process and consistently strive toward equality in the partnership, the chances for a successful outcome are greatly enhanced.

Researcher Reflection

What are some tips for merging traditional scientific research with the CBPR approach?

You could get up on your high horse and say, well, this is the way we need to do this because this is the best kind of science. And the reality will be, if you're going to stick with that, you're not going to have a project and nothing is going to get done. So, a lot of it is just being willing to realize that there is a difference between how science looks when you learn it in research methods and how it actually looks when you do it in a community. You have to be very creative about trying to come up with the best kind of designs that fit into real world situations with real world people. So, start at the end, start at the vision, and then work back from there. If you can agree on the vision, you can probably come to an agreement on the process.

Excerpted from a video interview with Gloria Eldridge, Ph.D., Associate Professor of Psychology, University of Alaska Anchorage

How Are All Partners Kept Informed of Process and Progress?

The ebb and flow that are common characteristics of human relationships create within themselves a somewhat fragile state. To maintain stability in the partnership, a strong infrastructure for open communication must be a priority from the beginning. This infrastructure forms a strong foundation that supports the following aspects of human relationships:

- Promoting and sustaining communication
- Ensuring and enhancing connectedness
- Respecting and accepting that each member's perspective is unique
- Maintaining and supporting commitment to meaningful work from all involved parties

One way to encourage community members to contribute is for all partners to engage in ongoing reviews of the research process as it relates to the principles of participatory research. It is important that:

- The scientific members of the research team monitor the distribution of power in the group.
- The community members monitor their own willingness to participate and contribute equally.
- All research team members carefully monitor their adherence to the strict ethical guidelines that were mutually created early on.

More ideas for communication options that work well for the CBPR process are presented in the first "How are day-to-day issues addressed?" question of this chapter.

Researcher Reflection

Who should help interpret study data?

As we completed each piece of the findings and summarized the results along the way, each section was shared both with the advisory committee and the telemedicine team—to review it, to make sure we had things right, and to interpret some of these findings. That really made a big difference particularly with the team who is responsible for the project, in their comfort level and having input into some of the subtleties of what those data suggested.

Excerpted from a video interview with Karen Ward, Ph.D., Professor and Director, Center for Human Development, University of Alaska Anchorage

The extent of the influence of a CAB on a research study will likely be dictated by the relationship between the principal investigator and the CAB. A PI who listens to CAB members and is willing to adjust the process based on their feedback will promote an effective, healthy CAB.

How Are Community Advisory Boards Maintained?

As noted in Chapter 3, forming a community advisory board (CAB) is an essential step in the CBPR process. However, simply setting up a board is not enough; the CAB must remain actively involved throughout the life of the project. Commitment from board members is not always easy to sustain, especially since some CBPR projects run for several years. It is essential to find ways to retain board members for consistency and effective functioning. The ultimate responsibility for maintaining an active CAB rests on the research team.

Valuing CAB Members' Contributions and Input

As discussed previously, a CAB is made up of individuals who are highly representative of community diversity. It is important for researchers to pay close attention to power differentials that occur naturally among CAB members, often reflecting each individual's relative status within the community. Each CAB member should see herself or himself as an equally contributing member of the group. Board members tend to be more committed to a CAB when they feel appreciated and perceive the CAB as a meaningful working group with an active and important role that is valued by the research team. Boards that meet only when specifically asked and have no active role in the project may take on a sense of non-importance, resulting in dropouts and frustration. Successful CABs are those with meaningful roles and important contributions, resulting in greater longevity.

Realistic Expectations

Researchers must be cautious to not exploit CAB members or make unrealistic demands on their time. Keeping a CAB meaningfully engaged without overworking its members requires several important skills on the part of the researcher. Despite the fact that CAB members are committed to the research project, they may struggle to fit the required activities into their day-to-day responsibilities and commitments. Researchers need to find ways to accommodate the unique situations of CAB members so they do not become resentful of the demands placed upon them. For example, meeting times may have to be changed on short notice when other commitments interfere. On the surface, this may not seem to be a major complication, but as changes and scheduling conflicts occur, timelines dictated by the funding agency may be affected. It is important for researchers to find ways to balance practical and personal aspects of the project.

How Are Major Changes in the 'Ground Rules' Addressed and Communicated?

Over the life of a community-based research project, adjustments to the ground rules are likely to occur. As previously discussed, changes in roles and responsibilities may occur in response to evolving community needs, strengths, and resources. Other changes will likely occur as partners reflect on newly generated knowledge throughout each phase of the project.

The Importance of Communication

Any adjustment to the process must be discussed and agreed upon by all partners. Small changes that are made early on can set the tone and provide experiential learning to help the group deal with larger issues throughout the project. Once the partners gain experience in group decision-making, future changes are likely to be handled more smoothly and in a manner that is acceptable to all.

When partners wrestle with change together, there is less likelihood that adjustments will lead to conflict or disagreement (ECPPRG 2006). Strategies for keeping communication open and ongoing include the following:

- *Regular discussions.* Regular, facilitated discussions should be scheduled during which partners can share grievances. Ongoing community forums provide visibility for the research team and allow community partners to remain informed as to process, change, and progress.

- *Specific agendas.* Specific agendas need to be created for all community events. These agendas should be circulated broadly and well in advance of the meetings.
- *Targeted discussion.* Assumptions of all partners need to be addressed early in the discussion process. Critical topics must be discussed in detail to be certain that individual and/or subgroup assumptions do not negatively affect the functioning of the partnership.
- *Monitor balance.* The distribution of power across partners needs to be carefully monitored to ensure balance among all partners.

Researchers must place high value on community input every step of the way, and ensure that their intentions and/or knowledge are not being imposed on the community. It is of great value and importance that the research project accurately reflects the realities of the community.

Conflict and Constructive Change

As stated earlier, conflict is virtually inevitable in any collaborative endeavor. Disagreements are bound to occur, and when handled appropriately, conflict can provide an opportunity for constructive change. Whenever a challenge arises and needs to be addressed, all partners are best reminded that the ultimate outcome of the CBPR project is to provide lasting benefit to the community. As all sides present their views of a difficult situation, the entire group remains focused on the shared goals of addressing the issue. Such shared goals include, but may not be limited to, all of the following CBPR objectives (ECPPRG 2006):

- It is important to know what each party wants—everyone needs to be heard.
- It is important to share common ground—the common goals that were established previously are reiterated.
- It is important that solution(s) to problems are fair to all—generate many options and then choose solutions collaboratively.
- It is important that the group not lose focus about its task—the team leader refocuses all members as needed.
- It is important to review all potential changes as they relate to power differences—all adjustments or modifications must be viewed through the lens of each participant.

With these common goals in mind, researchers can maintain the perspective that resolution of challenges drives good decision-making and healthy process adjustments. Partners who have a solid working relationship and mutual respect will likely approach and resolve conflict successfully.

Researcher Reflection

How do researchers and communities communicate their ideas of change?

For example, I might go into a community addressing HIV, but in that particular community, their bigger issue is sexual abuse of children, or hepatitis, or some other sexually transmitted disease that's all of a sudden reached critical mass and they want education about that. That's where you meet them at, and you tie the connection into what you're actually trying to study and you work around that. So it's sort of an agreement of ok I'll meet the community where they're at if they want more information on hepatitis. If they want more information on how to prevent child sexual abuse, then let's work that into this HIV Project. Because if you have a situation where you have a lot of people in your community who have hepatitis C, but nobody knows what hepatitis C is, but there's so much stigma around HIV, and it's a sexually transmitted disease and in the culture they don't talk about sex, and condoms are considered the government's way of creating genocide because people can't get pregnant with condoms, then you start with Hepatitis C. Then you start with Hepatitis B and how it's transmitted the same way as HIV and little by little you break down those barriers because really all they're interested in right now is Hepatitis C.

Excerpted from a video interview with Tracy Speier, MPA, Public Health Researcher, Anchorage, Alaska

Case Study 5.1

In response to a cluster of suicide attempts (one of which was success-ful) within a small community, university researchers approached a community with an offer of developing a suicide prevention program. Historically, the community had been closed to outside assistance; however, given the collective trauma experienced through the recent suicide and suicide attempts, community leaders and most community residents reluctantly welcomed the researchers. The researchers spent much of the first year developing community support for the suicide prevention project and establishing a local advisory board. Despite consensus-building efforts, some community residents continued to resent what they perceived as outside interference. Recognizing that full consensus would not be immediately attainable and with the sup-port of community leaders and most residents, the researchers moved forward with implementing the prevention project. To ensure that the project listened to all community voices, the researchers included on the advisory board an individual who was recognized as a leader from among those critical of the research project. Although the inclusion of this individual often made meetings challenging, over time, this indi-vidual came to recognize the value and importance of the prevention project for the community. As this individual's opinions about the proj-ect evolved, so did the opinions of community residents with whom he discussed the project. When the project was fully implemented and the researchers were gaining closure with the community, it was this indi-vidual who first asked the researchers to maintain an ongoing relation-ship with the community.

- What is the role of the Community Advisory Board in main-taining communication between researchers and community residents?
- How can the CAB be established to ensure inclusion of a diver-sity of community voices?
- What are other avenues through which community residents' agreement with a project can be maximized?
- What are creative solutions to including dissenters in ways that allow them to own the project and see its value without dis-counting their opinions and perceptions?
- How can researchers determine whether there is adequate com-munity agreement to move forward with a project?

Case Study 5.2

Early on, the research team identified community partners who, despite initial wariness and suspicion, committed to a research partnership. After initial growing pains, the group began to build cohesion and trust as the researchers became actively involved in community programs and events, engaging community partners both socially and professionally. Trust between the partners and commitment to the work and the partnership began to build over time. Prior to the start of project work, the researchers had obtained enough funds to take them through the first 2 years of the research. Due to the existing relationship that had been built between researchers and the community, the team identified community partners who, once invested in the work, sought out additional funding from national and local foundations, and from local, state, and federal agencies. The success of the community partners' seeking and receiving funding served to strengthen the partnership as funding from some of the sources was awarded directly to community partners, underscoring their roles as equals in the partnership and contributing to their confidence and investment in future community change (Metzler et al. 2003).

- How do members of the partnership benefit when responsibility is shared?
- How does sharing responsibility increase community capacity?
- What are the long-term benefits of increased community capacity in sustaining community change?
- How does sharing responsibility increase the community's investment in and ownership of the project and its results?

Case Study 5.3

A university research team joined an urban community in an effort to find treatment interventions for injection drug users with AIDS. Many of the partners were members of the local African-American and Latino communities. One very enthusiastic member of the outside research team, anxious to learn more about the community, spent time in households and community organizations, and attended many local community events. Eventually the researcher began to use language and gestures that imitated those of community members. Some community members strongly objected to her behavior, seeing it as a strategy to gain status or acceptance within the community. The team was able to resolve the conflict by holding open discussions about community culture, what it means to members of a group, and the importance of maintaining respect and coexistence of cultural differences within the partnership.

- How can individuals learn to respect cultural differences that exist among members of the partnership?
- What is the value of understanding your own cultural perspectives?
- How do researchers join a community without giving up their own cultural identity?
- What do community members expect from the research team?
- Why might the community value the cultural diversity the research team brings to the community?
- How is the project affected by a broad scope of perspectives, values, and culture?

Chapter 6
Evaluating the Partnership and Enhancing Future Successes

Upon completion of **Chapter 6: Evaluating the Partnership and Enhancing Future Successes**, the reader will be able to:

- Recognize and explain the importance of community input in the interpretation of data and dissemination of study results.
- Identify ways to successfully complete the study while sustaining the relationship with the community.

Introduction

After the work of data collection is finished partners should make collective decisions on the interpretation and dissemination of study results. During this final project phase, it is important that researchers remain true to the equity and respect for community partners that have been maintained throughout the project. Community partners may even be granted a "one-up" position in determining who "owns" the study data. The community often takes the lead in the interpretation and application of the results. Although publication in peer-reviewed journals is a goal of many traditional researchers, it is not necessarily the primary focus of CBPR researchers. Instead, the important aims of CBPR are to generate new knowledge, and make a lasting, positive impact on the community.

L.W. Roberts, *Community-Based Participatory Research for Improved Mental Healthcare*, DOI 10.1007/978-1-4614-5517-2_6,
© Springer Science+Business Media New York 2013

Chapter 6 focuses on completing the work of the CBPR project with the community, evaluating the process, and continuing the relationship. It underscores the importance of maintaining the partnership after the project is completed and describes how researchers can finish the work without community partners feeling abandoned. This chapter emphasizes the value of researchers maintaining a strong, healthy relationship with the community that extends beyond the life of the project. By conducting successful CBPR, and by building and maintaining a long-term, trusting partnership, the stage is set for future collaboration between the community and the research team.

Researcher Reflection

Why is it important to discuss dissemination throughout the CBPR process?

Think about that right from the very beginning and have that as part of your discussions. As you're setting up a project, ask yourself, What is the process for making decisions about how we will use the data at the end? Rather than assuming that we'll just do what we always do, we collect the data at the end, we analyze it, we write papers, we disseminate it. It's a more complicated process. I think you need to be thinking about it and talking about it all the way along. So you don't have any unfortunate surprises on either side.

Excerpted from a video interview with Gloria Eldridge, Ph.D., Associate Professor of Psychology, University of Alaska Anchorage

---

How Are Study Results Used in Ways That Are Acceptable to All?

When data collection is complete, and the research team prepares to analyze and report study results, it is crucial that community partners remain involved. Indeed, all final project work must be as respectful of the community as was true at all other times during the study. Community guidance during the interpretation and dissemination of study results is essential, which is contrary to the ways of traditional research. Community involvement during these final project stages contributes to results that truly benefit the very people responsible for generating the data.

In this final phase of project work, researchers allow community partners to take the lead in defining what study results mean to the community. It is the researchers' role to serve as catalysts to stimulate thinking among community partners, rather than imposing interpretations on them. The researchers' emphasis during this stage of CBPR is on process more than a predetermined outcome.

As community partners become involved in completing the study, they begin to think carefully about the links between process and outcome, and how study results can be applied to benefit their community in a meaningful way. By facilitating critical analysis, researchers can help community partners recognize the value of the work accomplished in the study, arrive at their own conclusions, and take positive community action based on those conclusions.

In keeping with CBPR principles, the community partners drive all decisions related to data ownership, dissemination of study results, and the use of findings. Their involvement at this stage can include all of the following actions and more:

- Commenting on and questioning study findings
- Creating interpretations that reflect the needs, culture, and values of the community
- Revisiting previous discussions about data ownership (although data ownership is discussed during this final phase of project work, it must also be part of the original research agreement negotiations and reviewed continually)
- Driving decisions about how study results are to be disseminated, if at all
- Discussing how to best use results to address the needs and interests of the greater community

Many communities expect or require complete ownership of study data and results, whereas others are willing to allow the research team to share ownership. Some communities are concerned about researchers using study results solely to further their own professional research careers, with little or no regard for the impact of published findings and interpretations on the community. These concerns are not unrealistic, as such occurrences have considerable presence in current and past published literature.

Ongoing Discussion of Dissemination Procedures

It is a good idea for research partners to collaborate on decisions regarding dissemination procedures in the earliest stages of project planning. However, even after such a path is determined and documented in writing, it is important that these decisions not be considered rigid or final. As with all other aspects of CBPR, dissemination procedures must be revisited throughout the life of the project, and may need to be adjusted as new knowledge is gained. This is especially true for community partners who may not have been fully aware of the implications of potential findings from the beginning. Early in project planning, some issues may not seem relevant or may not be anticipated. Such issues, once revealed, may greatly affect what a community decides about dissemination of findings. Further, if the focus of the study changes over time, community partners need to consider the effect of dissemination of study data on the larger community, particularly if unexpected or less than positive results are involved.

Discussions about study results must include a broad scope of community representatives to ensure that all community perspectives are considered. Also, the knowledge and findings to be disseminated to partners, as well as the community-at-large, must be communicated in language that is understandable by all and respectful of local culture and values. However, dissemination to the greater community does not necessarily approve revealing the findings beyond the boundaries of the community. The methods for dissemination to the community need to be chosen carefully. For example, it may not be appropriate to publish findings in a local newspaper in hopes of reaching everyone in the community. Once findings are in such a public domain, the research team loses control over where the findings may be distributed. However, other dissemination strategies such as organizational newsletters, videos, lay publications, or community meetings are methods to communicate results to the participating community while maintaining control over the breadth of dissemination.

Academic Researcher Issues

Many academic researchers involved in CBPR walk a fine line, as they may be conflicted between strict adherence to the principles of participatory research and their own professional development needs.

Among academics, some of the most frequently discussed barriers to conducting community-based research are the challenges associated with trying to achieve tenure and promotion. Most academic researchers are interested in publishing their study results in peer-reviewed journals (which often place greater value on traditional, quantitative research). However, participatory principles require researchers to consult with their community partners before submitting written work for publication. Researchers must be very careful to not publish any study results without the support of the community.

˙ In addition to professional development issues, community-based researchers often struggle with maintaining academic integrity and truthfully presenting results while respecting and valuing their community partners' interpretation of data and study results. Research team members hoping to become published should explore options that meet their professional commitment to increasing scientific knowledge in the professional community while still respecting the basic tenets of CBPR. For example, one alternative is to develop a manuscript based solely on the process of conducting the research project, without including the findings. In this fashion, other researchers become aware of study activities that may benefit other communities. Another option is to report the research findings without identifying the community. In instances in which community partners agree to make study results public, community leaders may be willing, and even eager, to assist with writing an article. No single answer exists for how to develop a dissemination plan that will work for all partnerships. Rather, each partnership must develop its own procedures to ensure that the dissemination of findings is mutually acceptable and, in the best case, mutually beneficial.

Much work remains to more fully develop and implement CBPR in mental health research and practice. Indeed, part of this work involves increased development of CBPR methodologies themselves, including identifying the essential components of CBPR in mental health research, and then evolving ways to execute these components effectively.

Ruth O'Hara, Ph.D.,
Associate Professor, Department of Psychiatry and Behavioral Sciences, Stanford University School of Medicine

How Is the Relationship Sustained When the Work of the Research Study Is Finished?

After the project is finished, researchers need to carefully ease out of the process—but not the relationship. CBPR principles require research teams to continue their commitment to community involvement and support of community needs beyond the work of the study. It is important to preserve the professional ties established with community leaders and organizations, as well as the personal relationships with community members. This is particularly true with groups in which members have felt exploited in the past by researchers who imposed their agendas on the community, and then abandoned it when their work was finished.

As has been stressed many times throughout this book, in any CBPR undertaking, one of the most essential activities is building, monitoring, and maintaining a trusting, equitable relationship with the community. For community members to gain trust in the relationship, they must be assured from the beginning that the research team places the highest value on community needs.

CBPR Trust-Building Process

As community partners experience the participatory process, they build trust in:

- The value their expertise brings to the work
- Their capacity to play an important and active role in the research process
- The reality that they truly have a valued voice in all aspects of the work

At the same time, the community builds trust in the researchers' promises to:

- Conduct research *with* the community partners, not *on* them
- Help develop community capacity to support and sustain community benefit and change
- Maintain the relationship that will extend well beyond the conclusion of the work of the research project

Researcher Reflection

How do you maintain relationships over time?

Maintaining contact, maintaining updates. On our community advisory board we provided periodic updates even when there were long stretches, like six months, when we didn't meet. But in terms of in-between projects, it's important to continue some connections so people not just remember who you are but know that you're still involved; that you still see their issues as important; and that you can be relied on. It's also important to give back, and so giving back can also be a way of maintaining these connections, such as giving presentations, holding work-shops, participating in grant writing. Reciprocation can be a very important way to maintain community connections.

Excerpted from a video interview with Inna Rivkin, Ph.D., Assistant Professor of Psychology, University of Alaska Fairbanks

How and Why Have Reflection and Debriefing Become Essential Activities?

CBPR is built upon a foundation of ongoing personal and group reflection that examines new information—which, in turn, is used to inform the cyclical process and produce new knowledge. Throughout the life of the CBPR project, reflection is viewed as an essential activity that focuses on both the process and the partnership, looking at what is working and what needs to be changed. It sets the stage for framing of all tasks, goals, and activities.

Ongoing reflection and debriefing by both the group and its individual partners are key to keeping the research study free from biases, respectful of community culture and values, and focused on creating real and lasting change. In particular, self-reflection is an important activity for members of the research team. Self-reflection encourages researchers to be introspective and to consistently hold up their personal beliefs, biases, values, and assumptions for critical analysis. Although all researchers bring some degree of personal influence to their work, ongoing self-reflection can help identify situations in which these personal influences might negatively impact the process or result in disrespect, judgment, or inappropriate action.

Writing in a journal and participating in group reflection with other research team members provide channels through which personal thoughts and feelings can be identified, monitored, and kept out of the research process. The following list offers some creative, helpful strategies for self- and group reflection, but by no means encompasses all possible methods for this type of evaluation (Taylor 1991):

- *Prepare a list of personal beliefs.* Prior to entering a community, researchers can create a list of their opinions and assumptions about the community and its members. As the work progresses, this list can be reviewed regularly to help evaluate whether these beliefs are influencing the work of the study or any aspect of the relationship between the researcher and community partners.
- *Keep a journal.* A journal or log can be kept throughout the research project. Entries are most useful if they include accounts of what the researcher has observed in the field, as well as individual thoughts and reactions that parallel the observations. Thoughts and reactions are generally written from a subjective, affective perspective to document the individual's personal reactions to the process. This journal is separate from, and serves a different purpose than, a researcher's detailed research protocol notes, which offer an objective account of the research process.
- *Establish a review panel.* Researchers may choose to solicit help from other mental health professionals to review data and provide feedback. This strategy can assist in identifying areas that need more attention or are being overemphasized at the expense of other important considerations. Feedback from review panels can call attention to results that may have been skewed, missed, or misinterpreted.
- *Form a community review panel.* A group of community members can be assembled to help with data collection, analysis, and interpretation and to assist with identification of errors of omission and commission not intended by the research team. Members of this group should accurately represent the diversity of the community. This review panel is most often independent of the community advisory board (CAB) discussed in earlier chapters.

How Is the Success of the Process Involved in Project Implementation Evaluated from the Perspectives of All Stakeholders?

In addition to personal and group reflection, ongoing process evaluation is necessary to ensure that participatory research principles are being followed. Such evaluation can involve review of the project's process, relationships, conflict resolution techniques, data collection systems, and more—providing new information that is timely, understandable, and useful. When partners collectively interpret the new information, process adjustments can be made that reflect this new knowledge.

CBPR process evaluation can be accomplished simply and inexpensively. It can take many forms, including, but not limited to, the following:

- Open discussions during regular meetings
- Face-to-face interviews with community members
- Online or paper surveys made available to the larger community

For example, the leader of the community advisory board (CAB) might interview board members between meetings to assess their satisfaction with the board's function and purpose. No matter what form it takes, frequent evaluation of both the process and the relationship contributes greatly to the success of the project.

Researchers should keep the following in mind when conducting CBPR process evaluations. First, it is important to begin the evaluation very early on and to continue regular evaluations throughout the life of the project. Adherence to the participatory process dictates that the research team and, at times, other interested parties review what is going well and what may need adjustment. All process evaluations should be heavily influenced by community perspectives. Outcomes must focus on elements that the community defines as important. Community representatives are well positioned to dictate the method used to collect information.

Numerous benefits result when much of the responsibility for process evaluation is turned over to the community:

- Capacity for decision-making increases when community partners own the evaluation data.

- Community involvement provides a method for ongoing communication about the research process, as well as a method to keep the research team accountable to the larger community.
- Significant involvement of community members contributes to the authenticity of the project and the likelihood that all aspects of the project truly reflect their situation. Although researchers may have specific ideas about how to measure the project's overall success, the community must have the strongest voice in naming the indicators of success that truly reflect the wants and needs of the community. Not only is it important that the community name the items to be evaluated, it must also develop evaluation methods that reflect local culture and values.
- Community ownership of process evaluation tools, methods, and results supports the participatory research principle of valuing local knowledge and experience, and it promotes capacity-building within the community.
- Communication is enhanced. Community representatives discover important information about the study and the partnership that can be communicated to the larger community.

Such active involvement increases the research team's accountability to the community in regard to process and outcomes. Open communication between those involved in the study and the community-at-large helps to ensure that the project focus stays on track and that the needs and wants of the greater community are being met. This is the fundamental purpose of community-based participatory research—to effect real and lasting change for the benefit of the community under study.

Researcher Reflection

Why is CBPR being done?

CBPR is not being done to advance a person's portfolio publications. It's a very different rationale for why the research is actually being done. And that it is benefiting the people who are the participants. They are no longer the "study subjects"; they aren't those people who are being surveyed or interviewed; they are all partners; they're collaborators in the research. And I think that those are positive aspects, that this is a changing way. The whole postmodern approach to science I think people are being to look at as a fact that we cannot just look at the science. I mean, numbers will give you the center of the bell shaped curve, but people live all the way out to the edges of that bell. So in order to get a sense, particularly if people at the edge are the people having some difficulties, that's where you want to focus your study. You don't want to look at what is the statistical norm; you want to look at what's outside your core. I think this is an exciting piece about community based research... that it's not that your average person has all these health problems; it's the exceptional persons who you need to have programs that focus on that exceptional environment.

Excerpted from a video interview with Carl M. Hild, Ph.D., M.S., Associate Director, Institute for Circumpolar Health Studies, University of Alaska Anchorage

Case Study 6.1

The study methodology involved participants completing question-naires and semi-structured interviews with the academic team. According to the research plan, the team decided to prepare a booklet of study findings to be distributed to participants as soon as the results were finalized. During the course of data collection, a number of participants indicated that they would like to meet with others who were involved in the project. They expressed a desire to reflect on the process and share their experiences with others. In order to facilitate this request, and to continue strengthening the relationship with the community, an initial, verbal sharing of research findings occurred in the context of luncheons held for the research participants. Approximately two-thirds of the participants attended the luncheons, which included social time, and a discussion of the research findings. Participants were invited to comment on, discuss, or challenge the findings, as well as offer alternate interpretations and their thoughts on ways to use the findings to benefit the community. These partici-pants became more invested in the work of implementing later pro-grams based on the research because of their heightened levels of personal investment, influence, and ownership in the work based on their increased participation.

- Who best represents the community perspective when inter-preting study results?
- How can study results best be shared with the community?
- How do you maintain scientific responsibility when interpret-ing study results while respecting community interpretation?
- Do individual biases play a part in community members' inter-pretation of study results?
- How do you interpret/recognize personal bias?
- When results are made public, how is the news managed?

Case Study 6.2

An ethical dilemma arose during a recent study of systematic and individual barriers experienced by visible minority workers in main-stream health agencies. One of the challenges in the study concerned the presentation of findings. During the collection of qualitative data, direct quotes were obtained from members of local racial minority communities about what they perceived to be acts of discrimination. When reviewing the data, institutional researchers were torn because they wanted to present an unbiased research perspective, but they felt that any commentary or analysis of the quotes and comments of study volunteers would contain elements of their personal values and perspectives. However, when study results are presented without researcher interpretation and analysis, readers of the research often feel that the work is biased and does not look at all sides of an issue. The assumption is that the work is poorly done and conclusions are not based on western standards. During data reporting, it became clear that one's race, gender, class, and sexual orientation affect data analysis and interpretation, and that reporting non-biased findings is often a fine balancing act between maintaining integrity, respect, honesty, and credibility.

- How can the interpretation of results reflect community perspectives and remain bias-free?
- Can scientific integrity always be maintained when the community perspective prevails in results interpretation?
- How do you respect community interpretation when results are made public?
- What issues might rise when articles are prepared for publication?

Case Study 6.3

At the end of a 5-year federally funded grant, a university-based research group and a small rural community came to the end of a project evaluating the effectiveness of a program designed to treat depressive disorders in women living in rural communities. Taking into account the planning and implementation phases of the project, this collaboration and partnership spanned approximately 7 years. At the end of the grant, the research group was forced to place its time and energy on newly funded projects and on seeking out additional funding sources to keep its doors open. However, the research group and the community leaders were very concerned about losing the partnership they had built over the years. In addition, the community had experienced measurable improvement in the health and wellness of its families, a success they attributed to the mental health program for women. Through brainstorming sessions, the researchers and community members decided to find ways of staying connected. The community contributed to the effort by continuing to collect programmatic data and providing permission to the research group to analyze the data and use them for publication purposes. The researchers contributed by giving the community opportunity to preview all research findings and provide consultation about the meaning of the findings in the context of the community's values and culture. Ongoing efforts were made to identify community mental health needs and apply for funding to secure services through pro bono work by the research team. Ultimately, another federal grant was funded for the purpose of preparing and submitting the original women's mental health program as an evidenced-based practice for rural communities.

Important Issues to Address

- What were the benefits to the research group in maintaining an ongoing relationship with the community?
- What were the benefits to the community to maintain an ongoing relationship with the research group?
- What obstacles could have gotten in the way of maintaining this relationship long term for both the researchers and the community leaders?
- In what ways did the research group show respect toward the community and utilize the community's expertise?
- How did the research group maintain the relationship even with limited resources and no funding? Why would they have done this?

Appendix A
Researcher Guide

Community-Based Participatory Research
for Improved Mental Healthcare

researcher guide

While there's no single blueprint for achieving success in a community-based participatory research (CBPR) study, following these general guidelines will help you establish a collaborative partnership with the community. Remember to continually hold the community input and perspectives in highest regard and to strive for respectful, equitable relationships with all community members.

Guidelines for Entering Communities

- Become involved. Establish roots in the community. Participate in community-sponsored events or volunteer time to local organizations. Contribute to community projects by collaborating with community-based agencies, clinics, health departments, or other mental health treatment providers on community health projects.
- Study social settings. Spend time with community members. Observe day-to-day activities. Engage individual community members in conversation, keeping in mind that much of a CBPR partnership rests on the social aspect of human relationships.
- Remain open to differences. Throughout all interactions, remain open to the similar/dissimilar, appealing/unappealing realities of community life, while reserving judgment of those realities and refraining from the impulse to change them. As the partnership is forming, differences of speech, dress, beliefs, and values must be accepted by both the community partners and the research team. Strive to understand the community's boundaries of acceptable values, behavior, and lifestyle.

Research Relationship Goals

- Maintain a truly participatory process. Remember that there is a distinct difference between community *involvement* (inclusion in the process) and community *participation* (equity of effort and influence).
- Uphold equity of power, cooperation, engagement, and respect between all partners.
- Build on strengths and resources within the community.
- Recognize that the research partnership is an ongoing co-learning experience.
- Appreciate the cyclic nature of participatory research; use new knowledge to direct the process.
- Empower and build capacity within the community.
- Build bridges with the community from *what is* to *what is possible*.
- Remember that community benefit must be the primary goal that guides all process decisions.

Communication Options to Ensure All Voices Are Heard

- Hold open meetings with facilitated group discussion to provide a platform to hear from many people.
- Offer a choice of small group discussion times to accommodate varying schedules.
- Provide a block of time during which community members can drop by to meet with the research team.
- Schedule one-on-one meetings between community members and researchers.
- Host town hall discussions to give less-involved community members a voice in the research process.
- Offer open-ended surveys or suggestion boxes through which community members may share opinions and views in anonymous fashion if they choose.
- Offer confidential e-mail communication with researchers.
- Provide the community with an online blog or bulletin board for input and discussion.

1

L.W. Roberts, *Community-Based Participatory Research for Improved*   121
Mental Healthcare, DOI 10.1007/978-1-4614-5517-2,
© Springer Science+Business Media New York 2013

Appendix B
Community Brochure (sample pages)

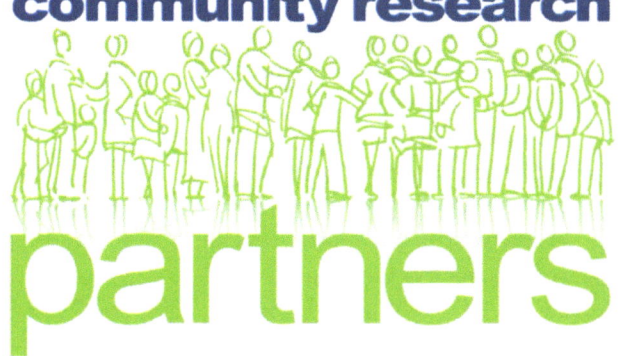

L.W. Roberts, *Community-Based Participatory Research for Improved* 123
Mental Healthcare, DOI 10.1007/978-1-4614-5517-2,
© Springer Science+Business Media New York 2013

Key questions to ask before joining a research study

- What is the purpose of the research?
- How will my community and/or I benefit?
- Where will the research take place?
- How long will the study last?
- What will my involvement be during the study?
- Are there any physical or other risks to participating?
- Will follow-up care be available after the study is over?
- How will the information collected be kept confidential?

Make your decision about volunteering when you are sure that you know all you need to know about every part of the research process. Also, if you have joined a research study and find that you have concerns or questions, it is your right to leave the study at *any* time, for *any* reason, without consequence or question.

What are the benefits of community-based research?

By working together, researchers, and community members share knowledge and experiences *with each other.*

When scientific research teams work closely with community partners, the study results are unique to the needs of the community.

Your involvement in community-based research will help develop solutions that fit the mental health problems that may exist in your life, or the lives of your family, friends, or fellow community members. The goal of a community-based participatory research project is to address unique community mental health issues, and to build skills and abilities within the community for creating and sustaining positive change.

> *Community members and the research team benefit equally by learning from each other.*

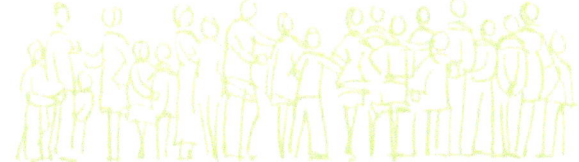

What can I expect from the research team?

You can expect that all partners are committed to the same goal – community benefit. Also, the scientific researchers will hold the opinions and contributions of the community in the highest regard.

Community-based researchers are committed to:

- Valuing and respecting the input and perspectives of community members
- Respecting the culture and values of the community
- Working to build community skills and resources
- Collaborating with community partners throughout the research project

Community members contribute their stories and life experiences... their thoughts and values... their understanding of community life... which are very important in understanding community needs.

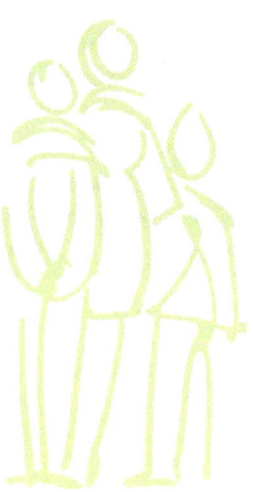

Appendix C
Facilitator Guide

Community-Based Participatory Research
for Improved Mental Healthcare

facilitator guide

guidelines for hosting community meetings

CONTENTS

L.W. Roberts, *Community-Based Participatory Research for Improved*   127
Mental Healthcare, DOI 10.1007/978-1-4614-5517-2,
© Springer Science+Business Media New York 2013

Facilitator Guide

Specific suggestions for meeting preparation and execution are as follows:

Prior to the meeting

Work with community partners to:

- Determine length, format, and roles of team members.
- Prepare and print a meeting agenda.
- Select meeting location(s), day(s), and time(s) that will promote participation among diverse, representative groups of community members and leaders.
- Make arrangements for community member transportation to and from meeting location(s), as necessary.
- Prepare a meeting evaluation instrument or strategy (e.g., short survey, large or small group discussion, comment forms).

Prepare/print meeting materials—all available in the Outreach Kit on the course website:

Note*: Terra Nova has endeavored to create community outreach materials that are suitable to a wide variety of audiences. But please consider the brochure, slide show, posters, and advertisement as entirely customizable. If you'd like to incorporate local artwork, terminology, or anything else unique to your study, you are free to use these layouts as templates, reworking them as you see fit.*

- Print the following materials (or order preprinted color copies by contacting Terra Nova Learning Systems at 650-391-9565 or info@terranovalearning.com):
  - Posters—Select from a variety of announcement poster layouts.
    - *Posters with "basic info"* These poster PDFs contain "editable fields" for customization of the welcome meeting description and entry of the meeting's location, time, and date, plus contact information.
    - *Simple poster*: This poster also contains editable fields for the meeting's location, time, and date, or the blank poster may be printed and this information entered by hand.

- Post in areas where community members congregate (e.g., community centers, health centers, schools, churches, libraries) or hand out, mail, or e-mail copies to community members and leaders.
- Consider posting information in less busy areas of a building (e.g., corridors that are less trafficked, rest rooms) to provide people with a more confidential viewing environment.
  - Community Brochures   Make enough copies for the maximum number of attendees expected at the meeting; use printing instructions in the box below. The brochure PDF contains an editable field on the back cover for entry of study information.
  - Community Resources List   Make enough copies for the maximum number of attendees expected. Consider preparing a list of local web and other resources to use as a handout at the meeting.
  - Community Slide Show   Consider printing the slides for attendees.

Guidelines for Facilitating CBPR Slide Presentation

Facilitator(s) should review the following slide-by-slide notes prior to using the CBPR Slide Presentation at the community meeting. These notes are not designed to be a speaker's instruction manual, but rather to be a guide that can be adapted for each user's unique presentation and interaction style. Recommended questions for discussion are provided at the end to assist the facilitator in inviting and encouraging group participation.

The CBPR Slide Presentation is designed to complement the community brochure that is included in the Outreach Kit. Brochures should be distributed prior to the start of the meeting, and may be referred to during the slide presentation.

The slides are available in either PowerPoint or PDF format. Facilitators are encouraged to customize the slide discussion based on project focus and, most importantly, community context, setting, culture, and values. Facilitators with PowerPoint software are encouraged to customize the slides with information about their project.

Slide-by-Slide Notes

Slide 1

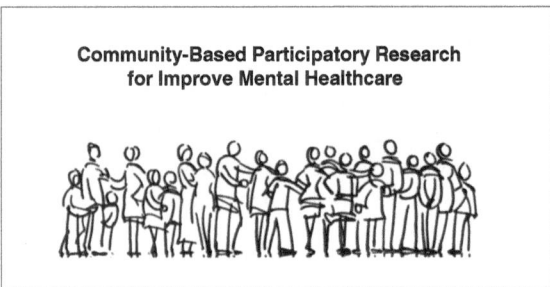

Welcome all meeting attendees; introduce members of the facilitation team as well as those who are assisting in other capacities.

Discuss the importance of the slide title: *Working together – Helping each other*. Stress to the attendees that the research will be conducted *with* the community for the <u>primary purpose</u> of improving the state of community mental health.

Talk about the critical importance of community input to the project. Communicate strongly that scientific knowledge alone is not enough. Input and guidance from people who are resident experts on community life is a critical ingredient in conducting research that specifically benefits unique community needs.

Slide 2

Welcome

You are a vital part of a community

- *Community* can include any setting where people come together with common interests, values, culture, perspectives, needs, etc.

- As a *community member* you are a "resident expert" on community life

---

Begin the presentation by recognizing that all attendees are members of a number of different communities, such as the following:

- Geographical (town, county, state, country, global)
- Racial/ethnic—sharing language, values, customs, culture, etc.
- Faith/worship
- Common interests (hobbies, sports, music, parenting, etc.)
- Community groups/local organizations
- Profession/work

Mention that these are just a few of the types of communities people belong to, but one thing is common throughout—members of communities have insights into community life that are critical to understanding and respecting that community's value, strengths, and needs.

Self-Assessment of Facilitation Skills

Answer these questions to help you reflect on the strengths of your facilitation style and to identify areas that may need improvement:

Active Listening—Hearing and understanding both subtle and direct messages.

- How well do I listen to participants?
- How attentive am I to nonverbal language?
- Am I able to hear both direct and subtle messages?
- Do I model effective listening and appropriate response?

Reflecting—Capturing the underlying meaning of what is said or felt and expressing this without being mechanical.

- Can I mirror what another person says without being mechanical?
- Can I restate what a participant has said with added meaning?
- Am I able to reflect both thoughts and feelings?

Facilitating—Helping members to express themselves clearly and to take action in a group.

- How am I helping participants work through barriers to communication?
- How much do I encourage audience interaction?
- How can I effectively attend to questions and group discussion while keeping the meeting on pace?

Empathizing—Adopting an internal frame of reference of community members.

- Are my life experiences diverse enough to provide a basis for understanding members?
- Can I maintain my separate identity while I empathize with others?
- How well do I communicate with others that I understand their subjective world?
- Am I consistently modeling appropriate empathy so as to promote empathy among community members?

Questioning—Using questions to stimulate thought and action but avoiding question/answer patterns of interaction.

- Do I overuse questioning as a facilitation style?
- Do I ask more "what" and "how" questions, and avoid asking "why"? ("Why" questions are often perceived as judgmental.)
- Do I ask open-ended questions to promote discussion and self-exploration?

Modeling—Demonstrating desired behaviors that facilitate group interaction.

- What kind of behavior do I model during group sessions?
- Can I model caring confrontations?
- What is the general effect of my behaviors on the group?

Appendix D
Meeting Poster (Sample)

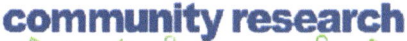

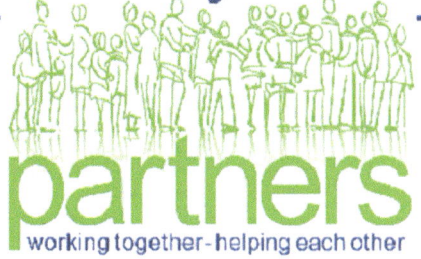

L.W. Roberts, *Community-Based Participatory Research for Improved* *Mental Healthcare*, DOI 10.1007/978-1-4614-5517-2, © Springer Science+Business Media New York 2013

Appendix E
Newspaper recruitment Ad (Sample)

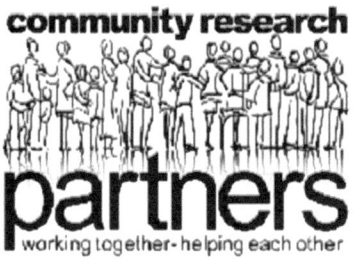

L.W. Roberts, *Community-Based Participatory Research for Improved*   137
Mental Healthcare, DOI 10.1007/978-1-4614-5517-2,
© Springer Science+Business Media New York 2013

Appendix F
Glossary

A

Affective
Outcome of or influenced by emotion.
Source: Berube, M.S. (Ed. et al). (2001). The American heritage dictionary (4th ed.). New York: Dell.

Anonymity
The state or quality of being unknown or unacknowledged. Anonymous information is that which an individual has disclosed with the expectation that the information will have no identifiers linked to the source and therefore will not be traceable back to the source in any way. Anonymity does not have the same meaning as confidentiality and is not interchangeable.
Source: Office of the Vice President for Research and Graduate Studies. (2006). SBC glossary. Retrieved from University of Virginia Research Web site: http://www.virginia.edu/vprgs/irb/sbs_glossary.html

Autonomy
Being able to make authentic, reasoned decisions for oneself. Self-determination.
Source: Roberts, L.W. & Dyer, A.R. (2004). Concise guide to ethics in mental health care. Washington, DC: American Psychiatric Publishing.

L.W. Roberts, *Community-Based Participatory Research for Improved Mental Healthcare*, DOI 10.1007/978-1-4614-5517-2,
© Springer Science+Business Media New York 2013

B

Beneficence
The commitment to act in a manner that brings about "good outcomes" or benefit to others. The duty to do good.
Source: Roberts, L.W. & Dyer, A.R. (2004). Concise guide to ethics in mental health care. Washington, DC: American Psychiatric Publishing.

Benefits
An expected advantageous outcome or result from an activity, project, or program.
Source: Terra Nova Learning Systems, LLC

C

Co-learning
A cooperative reciprocal educational approach in which participants actively share their knowledge, experiences, and expertise.
Source: Terra Nova Learning Systems, LLC

Collaboration
A mutually beneficial, cooperative work effort moving toward common goals and objectives. Information is openly shared and is dependent on mutual respect.
Source: Terra Nova Learning Systems, LLC

Commission
To do, perform, or carry out an act. In the context of health, an error of commission occurs as a result of an improper action taken. Examples include administering a drug at the incorrect time, performing surgery on the wrong body part, or giving a patient a transfusion with the incorrect blood type.
Source: Joint Commission on Accreditation of Healthcare Organizations. (2006). Glossary. Retrieved from http://www.joint-commission.org/

Community
A group of people, with existing relationships and shared interests, who interact in characteristic ways based on shared values to meet common needs.

Source: Schensul, J.J., LeCompte, M.D., Trotter II, R.T., Cromley, E.K., & Singer, M. (1999). Mapping social networks, spatial data, and hidden populations: Vol. 4. Ethnographer's toolkit. Walnut Creek, CA: AltaMira.

Community advisory board
(CAB) A group of individuals representing the local community that serve as a liaison between the researchers and the community at large; represent community opinion, culture, perspectives, and values in the research project; advocate for community rights; and facilitate full disclosure of information about the research project to the community. Membership of the CAB should reflect a true representation of the diversity of the community.
Source: Strauss, R.P., Sengupta, S., Quinn, S., Goeppinger, J., Spaulding C., Kegeles, S.M., & Millett, G. (2001). The role of community advisory boards: Involving communities in the informed consent process. American Journal of Public Health, 91(12), 1938-1943.

Community capacity
The skills and talents of individual community members as well as the associations and other resources of the community as a whole.
Source: Minkler, M. & Wallerstein, N. (Eds.). (2003). Community based participatory research for health. San Francisco: Jossey-Bass; and The Global Development Research Center. (n.d.) Urban capacity building. Retrieved from http://www.gdrc.org/uem/capacity.html

Community resource inventory
A written list of associations, organizations, and other individual and neighborhood-level resources available within a community.
Source: Minkler, M. & Wallerstein, N. (Eds.). (2003). Community based participatory research for health. San Francisco: Jossey-Bass.

Community review board
A review panel comprised of community members, stakeholders, and/or mental health professionals that review the proposed research to ensure adherence to accepted research ethics and human protections. The review board may also provide feedback to identify errors of omission and commission. Members of the review board should accurately represent the diversity of the community.
Source: Terra Nova Learning Systems, LLC

Community-based organization

(CBO) A nonprofit organization that helps community members obtain goods and services and helps to satisfy a community's physical, social, or economic needs.

Source: Schensul, J.J., LeCompte, M.D., Trotter II, R.T., Cromley, E.K., & Singer, M. (1999). Mapping social networks, spatial data, and hidden populations: Vol. 4. Ethnographer's toolkit. Walnut Creek, CA: AltaMira.

Community-based participatory research

(CBPR) A collaborative approach to research that equally involves all partners and recognizes the unique strengths and expertise that each brings to the process. CBPR starts with a research topic of importance to the community. The community and researchers generally share in the planning, implementation of data collection and analysis, and dissemination of research results.

Source: Minkler, M. & Wallerstein, N. (Eds.). (2003). Community based participatory research for health. San Francisco: Jossey-Bass.

Confidentiality

The obligation not to disclose information obtained from a person, or information gathered through observation in caring for a person, without the person's permission.

Source: Roberts, L.W. & Dyer, A.R. (2004). Concise guide to ethics in mental health care. Washington, DC: American Psychiatric Publishing.

Conflict

Prolonged opposition or disagreement between persons with opposing ideas, interests, or perspectives based on actual or perceived difference in goals or expectations.

Source: Terra Nova Learning Systems, LLC

Contextual

The circumstances in which an event occurs that determines its meaning. Putting a word or activity into a familiar context.

Source: Berube, M.S. (Ed. et al). (2001). The American heritage dictionary (4th ed.). New York: Dell; and Center for Research on Education, Diversity and Excellence. (2002). Glossary. Retrieved from University of California, Berkeley Web site: http://crede.berkeley.edu/tools/glossary.html

Contextualize
(See contextual)

Culture
Consists of the beliefs, behaviors, norms, attitudes, social arrange-ments, and forms of expression that form a describable pattern in the lives of members of a community or institution. Culture consists of group patterns of behavior and beliefs which persist over time.
Source: LeCompte, M.D., & Schensul, J.J. (1999). Designing and conducting ethnographic research: Vol. 1. Ethnographer's toolkit. Walnut Creek, CA: AltaMira.

Cyclical
A periodically repeated sequence of events.
Source: Berube, M.S. (Ed. et al). (2001). The American heritage dic-tionary (4th ed.). New York: Dell.

D

Data Safety Monitoring Board
(DSMB) An impartial group that oversees a clinical trial and reviews the results to see if they are acceptable. This group determines if the trial should be changed or closed.
Source: National Cancer Institute. Dictionary of Terms. Retrieved from http://www.nci.nih.gov/Templates/db_alpha.aspx?CdrID=44658

Debriefing
(1) To question formally and systematically in order to obtain useful information; to carefully review. (2) Giving participants previously undisclosed information about a research study following the com-pletion of their participation in the research.
Source: Office of the Vice President for Research and Graduate Studies. (2006). SBC glossary. Retrieved from University of Virginia Research Web site: http://www.virginia.edu/vprgs/irb/sbs_glossary. html and Terra Nova Learning Systems, LLC

Democracy
The principles of social equality and respect for the individual within a community or group and whose power is vested in the people.

Source: Berube, M.S. (Ed. et al). (2001). The American heritage dictionary (4th ed.). New York: Dell.

Dialogical co-learning

A collaborative and reciprocal learning process that involves a continuous exchange of information to develop mutual understanding and knowledge.

Source: Boyd, K.M., Higgs, R., & Pinching, A.J. (Eds.). (1997). The new dictionary of medical ethics. London: BMJ Publishing Group; and Visser, J. (2001, October). Learning communities: Wholeness and partness, autonomy and dependence in the learning ecology. Paper prepared for the meeting of the International Symposium on Learning Communities, Barcelona, Spain.

Dissemination

The systematic disclosure of information/knowledge—orally, in writing, or by electronic means—to potential beneficiaries to ensure that the information/knowledge is useful in reaching decisions, making changes, or taking specific action and is available to those who can most benefit from it.

Source: Southwest Educational Development Laboratory. (2006). National center for the dissemination of disability research. Retrieved from http://www.ncddr.org/index.html

E

Ecological approach

Views individuals as functioning within a complex system of social relationships affected by multiple levels of the environment, from immediate settings (e.g., family and peer groups, or school and work settings) to broad cultural values and norms. These relationships affect one another and guide interactions in local settings.

Source: LeCompte, M.D., & Schensul, J.J. (1999). Designing and conducting ethnographic research: Vol. 1. Ethnographer's toolkit. Walnut Creek, CA: AltaMira; and Berk, L.E. (2004). Development through the lifespan (3rd ed.). Boston: Pearson.

Efficacy

The ability to produce a desired effect or beneficial results. An examination of the impact of an intervention on the outcome under idealized circumstances.

Source: Sulmasy, D.P. & Sugarman, J. (Ed.). (2001). Methods in medical ethics. Washington, DC: Georgetown University Press.

Empathic listening

Being attuned to and conscious of what another person has to say, through both verbal and nonverbal communication, and recognizing that the other person's subjective reality may be different from one's own. Empathy involves identifying emotionally with another person and understanding the behavior of the other person in the context of his or her life (i.e., seeing the world through another person's eyes).
Source: Schensul, J.J., LeCompte, M.D., Trotter II, R.T., Cromley, E.K., & Singer, M. (1999). Mapping social networks, spatial data, and hidden populations: Vol. 4. Ethnographer's toolkit. Walnut Creek, CA: AltaMira.

Ethics principles

Principles that guide understanding and examining of moral life to create a coherent sense of what is good and right in human experience.
Source: Roberts, L.W. & Dyer, A.R. (2004). Concise guide to ethics in mental health care. Washington, DC: American Psychiatric Publishing.

Ethnicity

Self-designated membership in a sociopolitical group working toward maintaining its cultural and political presence, and to ensure protection, advancement, and access to resources for their members in a national system.
Source: LeCompte, M.D., & Schensul, J.J. (1999). Designing and conducting ethnographic research: Vol. 1. Ethnographer's toolkit. Walnut Creek, CA: AltaMira.

Experiential learning

A philosophy and methodology in which educators are purposefully engaged with learners in direct experience, focused reflection, and critical analysis in order to increase knowledge, develop skills, and clarify values. Learning through experience.
Source: Association for Experiental Education. (n.d.). What is experiential education? Retrieved from Association for Experiental Learning Web site: http://www.aee.org/customer/pages. php?pageid=47

F

Facilitated group discussion
Discussion led by a group leader or manager who is responsible for leading and coordinating the work of a group.
Source: LeCompte, M.D., Schensul, J.J., Weeks, M.R., & Singer, M. (1999). Researcher roles and research partnerships: Vol. 6. Ethnographer's toolkit. Walnut Creek, CA: AltaMira; and Lexico Publishing Group. (2007). Facilitator. Retrieved from http://diction-ary.reference.com/browse/facilitator

Frontier community
Isolated rural areas with extremely low population density, usually with fewer than six persons per square mile.
Source: Rural Policy Research Institute. (2006, November 22). Rural policy context: Frontier areas. Retrieved from http://www.rupri.org/resources/context/fa.html

G

Gatekeeper
Individuals who control access into a community, organization, group of people, or source of information.
Source: LeCompte, M.D., & Schensul, J.J. (1999). Designing and conducting ethnographic research: Vol. 1. Ethnographer's toolkit. Walnut Creek, CA: AltaMira.

Generalizability
Describes whether or not the research results can be extrapolated to or are relevant for a larger population, community, or group other than the one involved in the study.
Source: Health Compass. (n.d.). Glossary of terms. Retrieved from http://websites.afar.org/site/PageServer?pagename=HC_glossary

H

Harm

An undesired physical or psychological injury, damage, or loss which may be permanent or temporary.
Source: Berube, M.S. (Ed. et al). (2001). The American heritage dictionary (4th ed.). New York: Dell. Reworked by Terra Nova Learning Systems, LLC.

Hierarchical structure

(hierarchy) The organization of people, ideas, or things according to different ordered ranks or grades in an administrative body or system.
Source: Miller, G.A., Fellbaum, C., Tengi, R., Wakefield, P., Poddar, R., Langone, H., et al. (n.d.). WordNet: A lexical database for the English language. Retrieved from Princeton University, Cognitive Science Laboratory Web site: http://wordnet.princeton.edu

Humanism

A system of thought that centers on people and their values, capacities, and worth.
Source: Berube, M.S. (Ed. et al). (2001). The American heritage dictionary (4th ed.). New York: Dell.

I

Implicit

Implied or understood, though not directly stated or expressed.
Source: Berube, M.S. (Ed. et al). (2001). The American heritage dictionary (4th ed.). New York: Dell.

In vivo

An experiment or process that takes place within a living organism or cell.
Source: Terra Nova Learning Systems, LLC

Informed consent

The participant's formal consent or agreement to participate in a research study after being fully informed about the study design, process and uses of the data, risks and benefits of participation, and mechanisms for protecting confidentiality.

Source: LeCompte, M.D., Schensul, J.J., Weeks, M.R., & Singer, M. (1999). Researcher roles and research partnerships: Vol. 6. Ethnographer's toolkit. Walnut Creek, CA: AltaMira.

Institutional Review Boards

(IRBs) Committees mandated by the U.S. government that oversee the ethical treatment of human subjects in research.

Source: LeCompte, M.D., Schensul, J.J., Weeks, M.R., & Singer, M. (1999). Researcher roles and research partnerships: Vol. 6. Ethnographer's toolkit. Walnut Creek, CA: AltaMira.

Involvement

To be included in or a part of the activities of a group.

Source: Miller, G.A., Fellbaum, C., Tengi, R., Wakefield, P., Poddar, R., Langone, H. et al. (n.d.). WordNet: A lexical database for the English language. Retrieved from Princeton University, Cognitive Science Laboratory Web site: http://wordnet.princeton.edu

Iterative

Repetition of a process or action, cyclical or repeating.

Source: Terra Nova Learning Systems, LLC

J

Jurisdiction

The extent of authority or control.

Source: Berube, M.S. (Ed. et al). (2001). The American heritage dictionary (4th ed.). New York: Dell.

L

Lot system

A system based on chance or randomness.

Source: Terra Nova Learning Systems, LLC

M

Marginalized population
A social group of people excluded from the mainstream of society and placed legally or socially on the "margins" of society, thus limiting their resources for survival.
Source: Cushner, K.H., McClelland, A., & Safford, P. (2003). Online learning center: Glossary. Retrieved from McGraw-Hill Higher Education Web site: http://highered.mcgraw-hill.com/sites/0072486694/student_view0/glossary.html

Mutual
An interchange or reciprocal exchange of something between people (e.g., support, attention). A reciprocal relationship.
Source: Boyd, K.M., Higgs, R., & Pinching, A.J. (Eds.). (1997). The new dictionary of medical ethics. London: BMJ Publishing Group.

N

Noncoercive
To not force, dominate, restrain, or control forcibly.
Source: Berube, M.S. (Ed. et al). (2001). The American heritage dictionary (4th ed.). New York: Dell.

Nonmaleficence
The obligation to avoid doing harm to others.
Source: Roberts, L.W. & Dyer, A.R. (2004). Concise guide to ethics in mental health care. Washington, DC: American Psychiatric Publishing.

P

Participation
The process of taking an active part in or sharing control in an activity or task.
Source: Terra Nova Learning Systems, LLC

Pink collar
Employment classification that includes jobs traditionally considered female (e.g., waitress, librarian, nurse, secretary, florist).
Source: Terra Nova Learning Systems, LLC

Principles of participatory research
Participatory research core principles include the following guidelines:

• Research participants should actively set the agenda
• The research should benefit the community by providing tools to analyze conditions and make informed decisions on collective actions
• The relationship between researchers and community members should be collaborative and based on dialogical co-learning
• The process should develop the capacity of community people to appropriate and use knowledge from which they would be normally excluded
• The process should be democratic, enabling the participation of a wide diversity of people
• There should be a balance between research and community goals

Source: Wallerstein, N. (1999). Power between evaluator and community: Research relationships within New Mexico's healthier communities. Social Science and Medicine, 49, 39-53; and Freire, P. (1970). Pedogogy of the oppressed. New York: Herder and Herder.

Problem-solving skills
A set of skills that focus on logical, critical thinking and decision-making processes to solve a unique problem to a satisfactory solution.
Source: Terra Nova Learning Systems, LLC

Protocol
A precise and detailed research plan for scientific investigation describing the objectives, rationale, and methodology of the study.
Source: Terra Nova Learning Systems, LLC

R

Race
A local geographic or global human population distinguished by genetically transmitted physical characteristics and united by a common history, nationality, or tradition.
Source: Berube, M.S. (Ed. et al). (2001). The American heritage dictionary (4th ed.). New York: Dell.

Reciprocal relationship
A relationship in which all members give and receive for the purposes of mutual concern and benefit.
Source: Boyd, K.M., Higgs, R., & Pinching, A.J. (Eds.). (1997). The new dictionary of medical ethics. London: BMJ Publishing Group.

Research methodology
The overall plan for conducting a research project. The research design provides a flexible, working framework for the project.
Source: LeCompte, M.D., & Schensul, J.J. (1999). Designing and conducting ethnographic research: Vol. 1. Ethnographer's toolkit. Walnut Creek, CA: AltaMira.

Research partnership
The group of people collaboratively involved in a CBPR project, each of whom has an equal voice in the planning, implementation, analysis, and dissemination of the research. CBPR partners may include representatives from any or all of the following groups:

- Researchers (CBPR)—Outside scientific, academic, and institutional professionals who utilize the CBPR process to help guide the CBPR study, such as the principal investigator, research associates, statisticians, data collectors, interviewers, and other primary researchers.
- Research team (CBPR)—The entire outside research team, consisting of the above professionals plus additional physicians, psychologists, educators, social workers, mental health and substance abuse counselors, nurses, and other behavioral healthcare professionals.

- Community partners—People from within the community who contribute to the CBPR study by providing opinions and feedback and serve in a decision-making capacity, such as the following:
    - Community members* (including those living with mental illness, their families and caregivers, and the community at large)
    - Community leaders* (including representatives from local mental health agencies, government and religious leaders, and community advocates)
    - Local physicians and clinicians
    - Community advisory board (CAB) members

The term partner is used to describe any CBPR participant from the above groups.

*Typically, not every community member and leader will serve in an ongoing role in a research partnership. However, all members of the community at large are welcome and are encouraged to participate in a CBPR project to the degree they are able and comfortable. Please see Chapter 3 for suggestions on how to reach out to additional community residents.

Source: Terra Nova Learning Systems, LLC

Respect
The fundamental regard for the worth and dignity of a human person.
Source: Roberts, L.W. & Dyer, A.R. (2004). Concise guide to ethics in mental health care. Washington, DC: American Psychiatric Publishing.

Risks
An anticipated harm or possible loss.
Source: Boyd, K.M., Higgs, R., & Pinching, A.J. (Eds.). (1997). The new dictionary of medical ethics. London: BMJ Publishing Group.

Rural community
As defined by the Office of Management and Budget (OMB), a "rural" county is outside a metropolitan area and has a population of less than 50,000.
Source: Rural Policy Research Institute. (2006, November 22). Rural policy context: Metropolitan and non-metropolitan counties. Retrieved from http://www.rupri.org/resources/context/omb.html

S

Salient
Something that stands out is significantly noticeable, outstanding, or prominent.
Source: Terra Nova Learning Systems, LLC

Self-reflection
An activity of moral analysis about one's own impact, as well as how one's preferences, prejudices, biases, hopes, and concerns affect outcomes.
Source: LeCompte, M.D., Schensul, J.J., Weeks, M.R., & Singer, M. (1999). Researcher roles and research partnerships: Vol. 6. Ethnographer's toolkit. Walnut Creek, CA: AltaMira.

Social justice
The fair and equal distribution of benefits and burdens in society.
Source: Roberts, L.W. & Dyer, A.R. (2004). Concise guide to ethics in mental health care. Washington, DC: American Psychiatric Publishing.

Stakeholders
Individuals or groups who are affected by an issue and have a specific interest in the welfare of the community.
Source: LeCompte, M.D., Schensul, J.J., Weeks, M.R., & Singer, M. (1999). Researcher roles and research partnerships: Vol. 6. Ethnographer's toolkit. Walnut Creek, CA: AltaMira; and Terra Nova Learning Systems, LLC

Stigma
An attribute that is deeply discrediting to an individual or group and negatively affects their normal identity. Stigmatized attributes tend to evoke negative social feelings (e.g., fear, disgust) toward the individual or group.
Source: Boyd, K.M., Higgs, R., & Pinching, A.J. (Eds.). (1997). The new dictionary of medical ethics. London: BMJ Publishing Group.

Storming period
A normal and inevitable stage of team development in which the members begin to come into conflict, often over who in the group will hold power, how differences will be resolved, and role definement.

Source: Wheeler, J.C. (n.d.). What the heck is group dynamics? And what does it have to do with mastermind? Retrieved from http://www. grantmerich.com/articles.htm

Subjective

A mental act influenced by individual bias, opinion, or interpretation.

Source: Miller, G.A., Fellbaum, C., Tengi, R., Wakefield, P., Poddar, R., Langone, H. et al. (n.d.). WordNet: A lexical database for the English language. Retrieved from Princeton University, Cognitive Science Laboratory Web site: http://wordnet.princeton.edu/

Synergistic relationship

Relationship between two or more individuals or groups working together cooperatively so that the combined action achieves more than could be accomplished independently.

Source: Terra Nova Learning Systems, LLC

T

Tabula rasa

Latin term meaning a "blank or clean slate"; a fresh start; an opportunity to start over without prejudice.

Source: Miller, G.A., Fellbaum, C., Tengi, R., Wakefield, P., Poddar, R., Langone, H., et al. (n.d.). WordNet: A lexical database for the English language. Retrieved from Princeton University, Cognitive Science Laboratory Web site: http://wordnet.princeton.edu

Tempered

Finely adjusted, moderated, or attuned by adding a counterbalancing element (e.g., "criticism tempered with kindly sympathy").

Source: Miller, G.A., Fellbaum, C., Tengi, R., Wakefield, P., Poddar, R., Langone, H. et al. (n.d.). WordNet: A lexical database for the English language. Retrieved from Princeton University, Cognitive Science Laboratory Web site: http://wordnet.princeton.edu

Traditional research

A research approach in which the researcher applies formal, systematic procedures to obtain information through a disciplined and controlled process. Researchers base their findings on empirical observation and strive for information which can be generalized to other situations and larger populations or to generate further concepts and theories.

Source: (n.d.). Traditional research methods. Retrieved from http:// intranet.scpm.salford.ac.uk/studentintranet/dissertations/docs/traditional_research_methods.doc

V

Validity

The extent to which a measurement process (e.g., instrument or test) accurately measures what it is designed to measure.

Source: Phillips, J.J., & Stone, R.D. (2002). How to measure training results: A practical guide to tracking the six key indicators. New York: McGraw-Hill.

Volunteerism

Commonly characterized as nonfinancial work or service performed willingly for the purpose of mutual benefit to the volunteer and the recipient.

Source: Boyd, K.M., Higgs, R., & Pinching, A.J. (Eds.). (1997). The new dictionary of medical ethics. London: BMJ Publishing Group.

Vulnerable population

People who are unable to consent freely to participation in a research project because they may experience coercion, or be unable to understand the risks or procedures involved.

Source: LeCompte, M.D., Schensul, J.J., Weeks, M.R., & Singer, M. (1999). Researcher roles and research partnerships: Vol. 6. Ethnographer's toolkit. Walnut Creek, CA: AltaMira.

References

Adams A, Miller-Korth N, Brown D. Learning to work together: developing academic and community research partnerships. Wis Med J. 2004;103(2):15–9.

Association for Experiential Education: What is experiential education? Association for Experiental Learning Web site: http://www.aee.org/customer/pages.php?pageid=47 (n.d.). Accessed 8 Jan 2007.

Beecher HK. Ethics and clinical research. N Engl J Med. 1966;274(24):1354–60.

Berk LE. Development through the lifespan. 3rd ed. Boston: Pearson; 2004.

Berube MS, et al., editors. The American heritage dictionary. 4th ed. New York: Dell; 2001.

Boyd KM, Higgs R, Pinching AJ, editors. The new dictionary of medical ethics. London: BMJ; 1997.

Center for Collaborative Planning: Coping with conflict. http://www.connectccp.org (2002). Accessed 22 Sep 2006.

Center for Research on Education, Diversity & Excellence. Glossary. 2002. University of California, Berkeley Web site: http://crede.berkeley.edu/tools/glossary.html. Accessed 8 Jan 2007.

Cushner KH, McClelland A, Safford P. Online learning center: Glossary. 2003. McGraw-Hill Higher Education Web site: http://highered.mcgraw-hill.com/sites/0072486694/student_view0/glossary.html. Accessed 8 Jan 2007.

Department of Health, Education, and Welfare. The Belmont report: ethical principles and guidelines for the protection of human subjects of research. Washington, DC: OPRR Reports; 1979.

(The) Examining Community-Institutional Partnerships for Prevention Research Group. Developing and sustaining community-based participatory research partnerships: a skill-building curriculum. 2006. http://depts.washington.edu/ccph/cbpr/index.php. Accessed 28 Nov 2006.

Foulks E. Misalliances in the Barrow alcohol study. Am Indian Alsk Native Ment Health Res. 1989;2(3):7–17.

Friere P. Pedagogy of the oppressed. New York: Seabury; 1970.

The Global Development Research Center. Urban capacity building. (n.d.) http://www.gdrc.org/uem/capacity.html. Accessed 17 Jan 2007.

Health Compass. Glossary of terms. (n.d.). http://websites.afar.org/site/PageServer?pagename=HC_glossary. Accessed 12 Jan 2006.

Israel BA, Schulz AJ, Parker EA, Becker AB. Review of community-based research: assessing partnership approaches to improve public health. Annu Rev Public Health. 1998;19:173–202.

Joint Commission on Accreditation of Healthcare Organizations. Glossary. 2006. http://www.jointcommission.org/. Accessed 20 Dec 2006.

Katz J, Capron AM, Glass ES. Experimentation with human beings; the authority of the investigator, subject, professions, and state in the human experimentation process (compiled by Jay Katz with the assistance of Alexander Morgan Capron and Eleanor Swift Glass). New York: Russell Sage Foundation; 1972.

LeCompte MD, Schensul JJ. Designing & conducting ethnographic research: Vol. 1. Ethnographer's toolkit. Walnut Creek, CA: AltaMira; 1999.

LeCompte MD, Schensul JJ, Weeks MR, Singer M. Researcher roles & research partnerships: Vol. 6. Ethnographer's toolkit. Walnut Creek, CA: AltaMira; 1999.

Lexico Publishing Group. Facilitator. 2007. http://dictionary.reference.com/browse/facilitator. Accessed 17 Jan 2007.

Meslin EM. Final Report: White House Advisory Committee on human radiation experiments. The Hastings Center Report. Hastings Center. 1996. HighBeam Research: http://www.highbeam.com/doc/1G1-18825415.html. Accessed 06 Jun 2012.

Metzler M, Higgins D, Beeker C, Freudenberg N, Lants P, Senturia K, et al. Addressing urban health in Detroit, New York City, and Seattle through community-based participatory research partnerships. Am J Public Health. 2003;93(5):803–11.

Miller GA, Fellbaum C, Tengi R, Wakefield P, Poddar R, Langone H, et al. WordNet: A lexical database for the English language. (n.d.). Princeton University, Cognitive Science Laboratory Web site: http://wordnet.princeton.edu/. Accessed 13 Dec 2006.

Minkler M, Wallerstein N, editors. Community-based participatory research for health. San Francisco: Jossey-Bass; 2003.

Minkler M, Wallerstein N, editors. Community-based participatory research for health: from process to outcomes. 2nd ed. San Francisco, CA: Jossey-Bass; 2008.

Minkler M, Vásquez B, Tajik M, Petersen D. Promoting environmental justice through community-based participatory research: the role of community and partnership capacity. Health Educ Behav. 2008;35(1):119–37.

North American Primary Care Research Group (NAPCRG). Policy Statement on Participatory Research accepted at NAPCRG Annual Membership meeting, Nov 4–7.1998. http://www.napcrg.org/exec.html.

Office of the Vice President for Research and Graduate Studies. SBC glossary. 2006. University of Virginia Research Web site: http://www.virginia.edu/vprgs/irb/sbs_glossary.html. Accessed 13 Dec 2006.

Oldaker RA. How much do you know about the Amish? (n.d.). http://www.wvup. edu/Academics/humanities/Oldaker/about_the_amish.htm. Accessed 18 Aug 2006.

Phillips JJ, Stone RD. How to measure training results: a practical guide to tracking the six key indicators. New York: McGraw-Hill; 2002.

Roberts LW. Ethical dimensions of psychiatric research: a constructive, criterion-based approach to protocol preparation. The Research Protocol Ethics Assessment Tool (RePEAT). Soc Biol Psychiatry. 1999;46:1106–19.

Roberts LW, Dyer AR. Concise guide to ethics in mental health care. Washington, DC: American Psychiatric Publishing; 2004.

Rural Policy Research Institute. Rural policy context: frontier areas. 2006. http://www.rupri.org/resources/context/fa.html. Accessed 13 Dec 2006.

Rural Policy Research Institute. Rural policy context: metropolitan and non-metropolitan counties. 2006. http://www.rupri.org/resources/context/omb.html. Accessed 13 Dec 2006.

Schensul JJ, LeCompte MD, Trotter II RT, Cromley EK, Singer M. Mapping social networks, spatial data, and hidden populations: Vol. 4. Ethnographer's toolkit. Walnut Creek, CA: AltaMira; 1999.

Southwest Educational Development Laboratory. National center for the dissemination of disability research. 2006. http://www.ncddr.org/index.html. Accessed 13 Dec 2006.

Strauss RP, Sengupta S, Quinn S, Goeppinger J, Spaulding C, Kegeles S, Millett G. The role of community advisory boards: involving communities in the informed consent process. Am J Public Health. 2001;91(12):1938–43.

Sulmasy DP, Sugarman J, editors. Methods in medical ethics. Washington, DC: Georgetown University; 2001.

Taylor SJ. Leaving the field: research, relationships, and responsibilities. In: Shaffir WB, Stebbins RA, editors. Experiencing fieldwork: an inside view of qualitative research. Newbury Park, CA: Sage Publications; 1991. p. 238–47.

Traditional research methods. (n.d.). http://intranet.scpm.salford.ac.uk/studentintranet/dissertations/docs/traditional_research_methods.doc. Accessed 12 Jan 2006.

Visser J. Learning communities: wholeness and partness, autonomy and dependence in the learning ecology. Paper prepared for the meeting of the International Symposium on Learning Communities, Barcelona, Spain. 2001.

Viswanathan M, Ammerman A, Eng E, Gartlehner G, Lohr KN, Griffith D, Rhodes S, Samuel-Hodge C, Maty S, Lux L, Webb L, Sutton SF, Swinson T, Jackman A, Whitener L. Community-based participatory research: assessing the evidence. Evidence Report/Technology Assessment No. 99 (Prepared by RTI–University of North Carolina Evidence-based Practice Center under Contract No. 290-02-0016). AHRQ Publication 04-E022-2. Rockville, MD: Agency for Healthcare Research and Quality; 2004.

Wallerstein N. Power between evaluator and community: research relationships within New Mexico's healthier communities. Soc Sci Med. 1999;49:39–53.

Wheeler J.C. What the heck is group dynamics? And what does it have to do with mastermind? (n.d.). http://www.grantmerich.com/articles.htm. Accessed 14 Dec 2006.

Yankelovich D. The magic of dialogue. New York: Simon & Schuster; 1999.

Recommended Reading

Adler PA, Adler P. Stability and flexibility: maintaining relations within organized and unorganized groups. In: Shaffir WB, Stebbins RA, editors. Experiencing fieldwork: an inside view of qualitative research. Thousand Oaks, CA: Sage; 1991. p. 173–83.

Chambers R. Participatory rural appraisal (PRA): challenges, potentials and paradigm. World Dev. 1994;22(10):1437–54.

Chene' R, Garcia L, Goldstrom M, Pino M, Roach D, Thunderchief W, Waitzkin H. Mental health research in primary care: mandates from a community advisory board. Ann Fam Med. 2005;3(1):70–2.

Cochran P, Marshall C, Garcia-Downing C, Kendall E, Cook D, McCubbin L, et al. Indigenous ways of knowing: implications for participatory research and community. Am J Public Health. 2008;98(1):22–7.

The Collaborative Initiative for Research Ethics in Environmental Health. Dialogues for improving research ethics in environmental and public health. Conference report from the national conference. Providence, RI: Brown University; 2003.

Curd P, Winter S, Connell A. Participative planning to enhance inmate wellness: Preliminary report of a correctional wellness program. J Correct Health Care. 2007;13(4):296–308.

Denzin NK, Lincoln YS, editors. Strategies of qualitative inquiry. Thousand Oaks, CA: Sage; 2003.

Dick B. A beginner's guide to action research. 2000. http://www.scu.edu.au/schools/gcm/ar/arp/guide.html. Accessed 20 Jul 2006.

Digh P. Global literacies: lessons on business leadership and national cultures. New York: Simon & Schuster; 2000.

Ellis B, Kia-Keating M, Yusuf S, Lincoln A, Nur A. Ethical research in refugee communities and the use of community participatory methods. Transcult Psychiatry. 2007;44(3):459–81.

Fisher CB, Hoagwood K, Boyce C, Duster T, Frank DA, Grisso T, et al. Research ethics for mental health science involving ethnic minority children and youths. Am Psychol. 2002;57(12):1024–40.

L.W. Roberts, *Community-Based Participatory Research for Improved Mental Healthcare*, DOI 10.1007/978-1-4614-5517-2,
© Springer Science+Business Media New York 2013

Flicker S. Who benefits from community-based participatory research? A case study of the Positive Youth Project. Health Educ Behav. 2008;35(1):70–86.

Gagliardi A, Lemieux-Charles L, Brown A, Sullivan T, Goel V. Barriers to patient involvement in health service planning and evaluation: an exploratory study. Patient Educ Couns. 2008;70(2):234–41.

Garan NB. Community engagement: The magic potion. Paper submitted to the International Conference on Engaging Communities, Brisbane, Queensland, Australia. 2005. http://www.engagingcommunities2005.org/hone.html. Accessed 14 Oct 2006.

Gaventa J. The powerful, the powerless, and the experts: knowledge struggles in an information age. In: Park P, Brydon-Miller M, Hall B, Jackson T, editors. Voices of change: participatory research in the United States and Canada. Westport, CN: Bergin & Garvey; 1993.

Gibson, N. (Ed.). (1998). Responsible research with communities: Participatory research in primary care. Proceedings of the Respectful Research with Communities Workshop presented at the 1996 NAPCRG Annual Meeting, Vancouver.

Harding CM, VanPelt M, Ciarlo JA. Problems faced by consumers of mental health services out in a frontier community. Frontier Mental Health Services Resource Network, Letter to the Field No. 23. 2000. http://www.viche.edu/MentalHealth/Frontier/frontier.htm. Accessed 20 Jun 2006.

Henry ME. Debriefing sessions: opportunities for collaborative reflection. Kappa Omicron Nu Forum, 15(2). 2004. http://www.kon.org/archives/forum/15-2/Henry_2.html. Accessed 12 Oct 2006.

Horn K, McCracken L, Dino G, Brayboy M. Applying community-based participatory research principles to the development of a smoking-cessation program for American Indian teens: 'Telling our story'. Health Educ Behav. 2008;35(1):44–69.

House ER. Integrating the quantitative and qualitative. In: Reichardt CS, Rallis SF, editors. The qualitative quantitative debate: new perspectives. San Francisco: Jossey Bass; 1994. p. 13–22.

Hueston WJ, Mainous AG, Weiss BD, Macaulay AC, Hickner J, Sherwood RA. Protecting participants in family medicine research: a consensus statement on improving research integrity and participants' safety in education research, community-based participatory research, and practice network research. Fam Med. 2006;38(2):116–20.

Janecek Hartman J. Tribal college and universities return on investment (TCU ROI) conceptual model. 2008. PsycINFO database. Accessed 22 Apr 2008.

Kavanagh K, Absalom K, Beil W, Schliessmann L. Connecting and becoming culturally competent: a Lakota example. Adv Nurs Sci. 1999;21(3):9–31.

Keller PA, Murray JD, Hargrove DS. A rural mental health research agenda: defining context and setting priorities. J Rural Health. 1999;15(3):316–25.

Kelly PJ. Practical suggestions for community interventions using participatory action research. Public Health Nurs. 2005;22(1):65–73.

Kennedy Institute of Ethics. The national commission for the protection of human subjects of biomedical and behavioral research. Washington, DC: Georgetown University; (n.d.) p. 2–8.

Kirchner JH. Procedures and utilization of needs assessment in a rural area. J Rural Community Psychol. 1981;2(1). http://www.marshall.edu/jrcp/archives/Vol21/v21kirchner.htm. Accessed 16 Aug 2006.

Lee J. An examination of the effectiveness of community-based participatory research projects in producing intended health outcomes. 2008. PsycINFO database. Accessed 22 Apr 2008.

Leonard NR, Lester P, Rotheram-Borus MJ, Mattes K, Gwadz M, Ferns B. Successful recruitment and retention of participants in longitudinal behavioral research. AIDS Educ Prev. 2003;15(3):269–81.

Loftin W, Barnett S, Summers Bunn P, Sullivan P. Recruitment and retention of rural African Americans in diabetes research. Diabetes Educ. 2005;31(2):251–9.

Macaulay A, Commanda LE, Freeman WL, Gibson N, McCabe ML, Robbings CM, Twohig PL. Participatory research maximizes community and lay involvement. Br Med J. 1999;319:774–8.

Macaulay AC, Commanda LE, Freeman WL, McCabe ML, Robbins CM, Twohig PL. Responsible research with communities: participatory research in primary care (N. Gibson, editor). Policy statement on participatory research accepted at NAPCRG Annual Membership meeting, Montreal. 1998. http://www.nap-crg.org/responsibleresearch.pdf. Accessed 27 Oct 2006.

Maguire P. Doing participatory research: a feminist approach. Amherst, MA: University of Massachusetts, Center for International Education; 1987.

Mendel P, Meredith L, Schoenbaum M, Sherbourne C, Wells K. Interventions in organizational and community context: a framework for building evidence on dissemination and implementation in health services research. Admin Pol Ment Health Ment Health Serv Res [serial online]. 2008;35(1):21–37.

Mihesuah DA. Suggested guidelines for institutions with scholars who conduct research on American Indians. Am Indian Cult Res J. 1993;17(3):131–9.

Minkler M. Ethical challenges for the outside researcher in community-based participatory research. Health Educ Behav. 2004;31(6):684–97.

Minkler M, Fadem P, Perry M, Blum K, Moore L, Rogers J. Ethical dilemmas in participatory action research: a case study from the disability community. Health Educ Behav. 2002;29(1):14–29.

Mohatt G, Rasmus S, Thomas L, Allen J, Hazel K, Marlatt G. Risk, resilience, and natural recovery: a model of recovery from alcohol abuse for Alaska natives. Addiction. 2008;103(2):205–15.

The National Commission for the Protection of Human Subjects of Biomedical and Behavioral Research. The Belmont report: Ethical principles and guidelines for the protection of human subjects of research. U.S. Department of Health, Education, and Welfare. 1979. http://www.tarleton.edu/~grants/BelmontReport.pdf. Accessed 17 Jun 2006.

Nyden P, Wiewel W. Collaborative research: harnessing the tensions between researcher and practitioner. Am Sociol. 1992;23(4):43–55.

O'Fallon LR, Tyson FL, Dearry A. (Eds.). Successful models of community-based participatory research. Final report of a meeting hosted by the National Institute of Environmental Health Sciences, Washington, DC, p. 29–31.

Parasyn CL. Aharenmen! Who better understand a community than those who live in it! Paper submitted to the International Conference on Engaging

Communities, Brisbane, Queensland, Australia. 2005. http://www.engaging-communities2005.org/hone.html. Accessed 4 Oct 2006.

Portman TAA, Dewey D. Revisiting the spirit: a call for research related to rural Native Americans. J Rural Community Psychol. 2003;E6(1). http://www.marshall.edu/jrcp/E6one_Portman.htm. Accessed 7 Jun 2004.

Rearich E. Amish culture and healthcare. J Undergraduate Nurs Scholarship. 2003. The University of Arizona College of Nursing Web site: http://juns.nursing.arizona.edu/articles/Fall%202003/rearick.htm. Accessed 7 Nov 2006.

Roberts LW, Battaglia J, Smithpeter M, Epstein RS. An office on main street: health care dilemmas in small communities. Hastings Cent Rep. 1999;29(4):28–37.

Rosen R, Digh P, Singer M, Phillips C. Global literacies: lessons on business leadership and national cultures. New York: Simon & Schuster; 2000.

Seng J. Praxis as a conceptual framework for participatory research in nursing. Adv Nurs Sci. 1998;20(4):37–48.

Shaffir WB, Stebbins RA, editors. Experiencing fieldwork: an inside view of qualitative research. Newbury Park, CA: Sage; 1990.

Sixsmith J, Boneham M, Goldring JE. Accessing the community: gaining insider perspectives from the outside. Qual Health Res. 2003;13(4):578–89.

Sohng S. Participatory research and community organizing. A working paper presented at The New Social Movement and Community Organizing Conference, University of Washington, Seattle. 1995.

Starhawk. Truth or dare: encounters with power, authority, and mystery. San Francisco: HarperCollins; 1987.

Stoecker RR. Are academics irrelevant? Roles for scholars in participatory research. Am Behav Sci. 1999;42(5):840–54.

Stoecker RR. Research methods for community change: a project-based approach. Thousand Oaks, CA: Sage; 2005.

Wellons MF, Lewis CE, Schwartz SM, et al. Racial differences in self-reported infertility and risk factors for infertility in a cohort of black and white women: The CARDIA Women's Study. Fertil Steril. 2008;90(5):1640–8.

Whitener L. Research reviews – rural mental health care. J Rural Health. 1996;12(3):235–39.

Whitmore R. Final assessment paper. 2000. http://www.msu.edu/~prnetwrk/ronprclassfinal.doc. Accessed 6 Oct 2006.

Whyte WF. Street corner society. Chicago: University of Chicago Press; 1981.

Wiewel W. Harvard on Halsted Street: dilemmas of neighborhood advocacy in academia. Paper presented at the annual meeting of the Association of Collegiate Schools of Planning, Atlanta. 1985.

Wood GS, Judikis JS. Conversations on community theory. West Lafayette, IN: Purdue University Press; 2002.

Index